THE SOUTH BEACH HEART PROGRAMME

THE SOUTH BEACH HEART PROGRAMME

THE 4-STEP PLAN THAT CAN SAVE YOUR LIFE

Dr Arthur Agatston

Author of the No. 1 *New York Times* Bestseller *The South Beach Diet*

RODALE

This edition first published in 2007 by
Rodale International Ltd
7–10 Chandos Street
London
W1G 9AD

The moral right of Dr Arthur Agatston to be identified as author of this work has been
asserted in accordance with the Copyright, Designs and Patents Act of 1988.

Illustrations by Lisa Clark
Photographs by Mitch Mandel/Rodale Images
Book design by Carol Angstadt

Printed and bound in the UK by CPI Bath using acid-free paper from sustainable sources.

1 3 5 7 9 8 6 4 2

A CIP record for this book is available from the British Library.

ISBN 978-1-4050-9547-1

This paperback edition distributed to the book trade by Pan Macmillan Ltd.

UK medical consultant: Dr Julian Halcox
An expert in preventive cardiology, Julian Halcox specializes in the treatment and prevention
of coronary artery disease. In addition to his clinical work, Dr Halcox conducts a productive
programme of original research, largely funded by the British Heart Foundation, into the
development of coronary artery disease including the role of stem cells in early arterial disease.
He works as a Consultant Cardiologist at University College London Hospitals, Great Ormond
Street Hospital for Children and in private practice.

Notice
This book is intended as a reference volume only, not as a medical manual. The information
given here is designed to help you make informed decisions about your health. It is not
intended as a substitute for any treatment that may have been prescribed by your doctor. If you
suspect that you have a medical problem, we urge you to seek competent medical help.

The information in this book is meant to supplement, not replace, proper exercise training.
All forms of exercise pose some inherent risks. The editors and publisher advise readers to take
full responsibility for their safety and know their limits. Before practising the exercises in this
book, be sure that your equipment is well-maintained, and do not take risks beyond your level
of experience, aptitude, training and fitness. The exercise and dietary programmes in this
book are not intended as a substitute for any exercise routine or dietary regime that may have
been prescribed by your doctor. As with all exercise and dietary programmes, you should get
your doctor's approval before beginning.

Mention of specific companies, organizations or authorities in this book does not imply
endorsement by the author or publisher, nor does mention of specific companies, organizations or authorities imply that they endorse this book, its author or the publisher.

Internet addresses and telephone numbers given in this book were accurate at the time it
went to press.

To all the doctors who have pioneered,

believed in, and practised the prevention

revolution in cardiology.

And, as always, to my wife, Sari.

CONTENTS

PART

2

THE SOUTH BEACH HEART PROGRAMME

STEP 1

STEP 2

STEP 3

STEP 4

FOREWORD

The *South Beach Heart Programme* is based on a huge body of research in cardiology produced by thousands of brilliant doctors and investigators over many years. Thanks to these efforts, I believe we have reached a point where the great majority of heart attacks and strokes can be prevented.

I want to acknowledge in particular those thought leaders who have influenced my own understanding of coronary artery disease and its application in my everyday practice of preventive cardiology. Some are friends and collaborators, some are acquaintances, and some I know only through their writings and lectures. Naturally, I am concerned about unintentional omissions, and I apologize for these in advance.

As I relate later in this book, I first became excited about the potential for preventing heart attacks when I began attending the lectures of Dr William Castelli, the director of the ongoing Framingham Heart Study from 1979 to 1995. Doctors and the public owe a debt of gratitude to everyone involved in the Framingham study. Not only did data from Framingham allow investigators to pioneer the concept of cardiac risk factors, it continues to be an invaluable resource for doctors and researchers interested in the prevention of heart disease.

Once my interest in prevention was established, I learned more about cholesterol lipids and the potential of the early statin drugs from the lectures and writings of Drs Antonio Gotto, John LaRosa, David Waters and many others.

Thinking about who would be the best candidates for taking statins to lower their cholesterol levels stimulated my interest in the potential of noninvasive coronary artery imaging to detect the degree of risk for heart attack. With the close collaboration of Dr Warren Janowitz and the late David King of the then Imatron Corporation and the advice and support of Dr Manuel Viamonte, we developed the noninvasive heart scan for early detection of the extent of atherosclerosis. We were encouraged and helped early on by a group of fabulous doctors we called the Calcium Club, since our work was focused on detecting and quantifying coronary artery calcium as an indicator of coronary atherosclerosis. Included in this group were Drs John Rumberger, Patrick Sheedy, Bruce Brundage, Stuart Rich, Alan Guerci, Yadon Arad, Robert Detrano and Tracy Callister.

Over the years, many more doctors became important players in the development of noninvasive coronary imaging, leading up to recent advances in developing the noninvasive angiogram. These include Drs Stephan Achenbach, Allen Taylor, Paolo Raggi, Harvey Hecht, Daniel Rader, James Ehrlich, Leslie Shaw, George T. Kondos, Philip Greenland and Daniel Berman. More recently, Drs Michael Poon and Jack Ziffer taught me a great deal about the potential of the noninvasive angiogram.

While many researchers around the world contributed to the new 'healing' model of coronary disease that you will learn about in this book, Dr Valentin Fuster became the leader in research and teaching in this area. His lectures opened my eyes to the fact that the old 'plumbing' model of heart disease was simply wrong. I was also influenced by the important research of Drs Michael Davies, Erling Falk, William Roberts, Spencer King, Robert Bonow, Richard Devereux and Seymour Glagov, which helped to define the mechanisms of the progression of atherosclerosis.

In recent years, Drs Peter Libby, Robert Vogel, George Diamond, Eric Topol, Steven Nissen, James Forrester and Carl Pepine have elegantly explained the important role of our artery walls in preventing heart attacks. And Dr Richard Conti has been a tireless educator of cardiologists around the world.

The application of prevention strategies in reversing heart disease was first demonstrated by the late Dr David Blankenhorn. Drs B. Greg Brown, P. K. Shah, Dean Ornish and Lance Gould all impressed me with research showing that coronary disease could be halted and even reversed. And Drs Kenneth Cooper and Steven N. Blair taught me much about the role of exercise in cardiac health.

From 1997 until the present, my friend Dr Ted Feldman has held an annual symposium in Miami, Florida, that has brought together many of the leaders in the field of cardiac prevention. Drs Nanette Wenger (a pioneer in women's health), Fred Pashkow, George Diamond and Randy

Martin are among the symposium faculty who have taught me a great deal.

Once I began using the heart scan to detect atherosclerosis, it became particularly important for me to learn how to reverse the coronary disease I was seeing. It was at this time that I began to learn the importance of advanced blood testing from the lectures of Dr H. Robert Superko. From the work of Dr Paul Ridker, I became aware of the contribution of inflammation to coronary artery disease and the best ways to test for it.

My years at Mount Sinai Medical Center in Miami Beach, Florida, were enriched by the arrival of Drs Gervasio Lamas, Eric Lieberman and Francisco Lopez-Jiminez in the early 1990s; all became important collaborators in my research. They were also great teachers who advanced my understanding of the power and pitfalls of the clinical trial.

Learning of the existence and significance of the metabolic syndrome contributed to my understanding of how recent, disturbing trends in the Western lifestyle – mainly less exercise and poor diet – have led to our epidemics of obesity, diabetes and other chronic diseases. While it was Dr Gerald Reaven who first characterized the metabolic syndrome as an entity in 1988, I became aware of its importance through the teaching of Dr Ronald Goldberg of the University of Miami Miller School of Medicine's Diabetes Institute. In addition, the lectures and writings of Drs Scott Grundy and Steven Hafner greatly advanced my understanding in this area.

I have learned a great deal about nutrition from Dr Walter Willett and his colleagues at the Harvard School of Public Health; they have done more to create the present consensus on the principles of good nutrition than any other research group. The research and writings of Drs David Jenkins, David Ludwig and Jennie Brand-Miller have taught me the nutritional importance of the glycaemic index.

Finally, my interest in the history of diet, going all the way back to the era of the hunter-gatherer, has given me important insights into how we should be eating today. In this area, I have learned a great deal from the research and writings of Drs Loren Cordain and S. Boyd Eaton.

Again, I want to thank all those who have participated in the prevention revolution in cardiac care. I am confident that their work will continue to lead to better health and better lives for us all.

ACKNOWLEDGEMENTS

The *South Beach Heart Programme* is a book that I have wanted to write for many years because I believe so strongly in its message. A great many people have played roles in its creation, including numerous medical colleagues whom I thank separately in my Foreword. I also owe a great debt to my patients, who have been the inspiration for this book and who are living proof that preventive cardiology works. A special thanks to those who allowed me to use their stories. Except for Dr Ted Feldman, I have intentionally changed their names and some of the details to protect their privacy. I would also like to thank my nurse practitioner, Clarissa Gregory, and my physician's assistant, Xi Zhu, for their critique of the manuscript. In addition, my executive assistant, Ariel Rodriguez, has done an incredible job of helping me balance clinical, educational, research and writing responsibilities.

At Rodale, I would like to thank Liz Perl and Cindy Ratzlaff for their continuing enthusiasm and support. I would also like to thank Rodale art director Carol Angstadt, photographer Mitch Mandel, photo editor Marc Sirinski and project editor Hope Clarke for their work on the book.

I was particularly lucky to have two fabulous editors at Rodale, whose contributions, including their friendship, have been invaluable to this project. Margot Schupf was always available with expert advice, counsel and support. Marya Dalrymple was tireless in keeping our work on the right track. Despite having to be a taskmaster at times, Marya was always a pleasure and made a lot of hard work enjoyable.

I am also grateful to Margo Lowry of the South Beach Diet partnership for her incisive wisdom and constant support and to Marie Almon, my nutrition director, who advises my patients daily on the benefits of a heart-healthy diet.

In addition, I want to especially thank my attorney and friend, Andy Hall, whose advice, legal and otherwise, I always value; my accountant, Tim Devlin, who gave me a better understanding of the tax and economic implications of various health insurance plans and savings accounts; and Kris Belding, my trainer, who helped me develop my exercise philosophy and who works hard to keep my core and my heart in shape. Special thanks also goes to Alice McGillion and Lori Ferme of Rubenstein Communications for their help in spreading the word about good health and prevention.

Finally, there has been no bigger champion for this book and for my work than my wife, Sari, who has had to listen to me talk about preventing heart attacks and strokes for more than 25 years and who has inspired me to persist in advancing the prevention message. She is also my third editor and as such has made important contributions to this book. And, as always, I want to thank my sons, Evan and Adam, for their uninhibited and constructive criticism.

PART
1

No More
Heart Attacks
and Strokes

1

You Don't Have to Have a Heart Attack!

Imagine a world in which heart attacks are rare and death from a premature heart attack is virtually unknown – a thing of the past. Imagine a world in which heart disease is detected so early and so accurately – and treated so effectively – that very few people will ever need to be subjected to invasive and expensive procedures such as angioplasty or coronary bypass surgery. Imagine a world in which we can confidently look forward to healthy and productive lives free from the threat of heart attacks and strokes.

You may be thinking, 'My kids or grandchildren might be lucky enough to live in such a world, but this isn't going to happen in my lifetime.'

If that's what you're thinking, you're wrong.

The exciting news is that we now have the knowledge and ability to prevent the great majority of heart attacks and strokes. We can save hundreds of thousands of lives each year – maybe even yours. I'm not talking about what we will be able to do 10 years from now, or even 5 years from now. I'm talking about what we can do *right now*. What's even more remarkable is the fact that *right now* we have noninvasive – no cutting, no pain, no recovery required – diagnostic techniques that can identify people who are at high risk for developing coronary artery disease (or CAD), so that they can be treated early. We also have highly effective treatments, including medications and lifestyle changes, that can reverse damage to the heart's arteries without requiring patients to go under the knife. These treatments are simple and inexpensive when compared to angioplasty or bypass surgery.

I know this is true because I prescribe them every day in my medical practice. Many of you may know me as the doctor who created the South Beach Diet, but I am an *accidental* diet doctor. For nearly 30 years, I have been a cardiologist – a specialist in disorders of the heart – and for more than 20 years, I've been an associate professor at the University of Miami Miller School of Medicine at Mount Sinai. Much of my medical career has been devoted to noninvasive cardiac imaging, the technology that allows us to get detailed pictures of the heart and coronary arteries from *outside* the body. If you have ever had a heart scan – either a computed tomography (CT) scan or an electron beam tomography (EBT) scan – you were probably given a *Calcium Score* as part of your test results. That measure of coronary calcium is often referred to as the *Agatston Score*, and the method for calcium screening is called the *Agatston Method*. Both come from my early work with my colleague Dr Warren Janowitz, developing a method of imaging plaque-clogged arteries that can be employed years before heart attack symptoms occur. In fact, the diagnosis and prevention of heart disease has been my focus and passion throughout my professional life.

A Passion for Prevention

Today, an unbelievable 66.5 per cent of Americans are either overweight or obese, and 40 per cent of those over the age of 40 are prediabetic. Nearly 21 million Americans actually have diabetes, and that number is growing daily. What's more, we are exporting our epidemics of obesity, prediabetes and diabetes to the rest of the world at an alarming rate. As many as 300 million people worldwide have prediabetes and in the UK it is estimated that 3 million people will have type 2 diabetes by 2010. People who have these conditions, which are largely due to poor diet and lifestyle habits, are prime candidates for heart disease.

I developed the South Beach Diet to help my patients lose weight, improve their blood chemistries, and avoid becoming diabetic. It was a piece of the prevention puzzle and it worked. Thanks to the worldwide success of my first book, I have been given the unique and wonderful opportunity to help change the way people eat. And while I am thrilled that millions of people around the world are following the South Beach Diet, I have an even more ambitious agenda.

My goal in writing *The South Beach Heart Programme* is to speed the pace of the cardiac prevention revolution currently taking place in this country and elsewhere in the West.

I believe that one of the great failings in medical practice today is that cardiovascular disease is not diagnosed and treated in its earliest stages. Every time I hear that someone has died of a 'sudden heart attack', I can't help but think that it shouldn't have happened. A life could have been saved if the victim had just had the benefit of the latest diagnostic techniques and medical treatments.

The South Beach Heart Programme is based on these cutting-edge tools, which are currently being used by prevention-oriented cardiologists. It shows you how to make the most of these advances, while improving your diet and lifestyle as well.

Heart Attacks Can Be Prevented

From the moment I graduated from medical school, I had a great interest in preventing heart disease, but I didn't know how. That changed with the development of cholesterol-lowering drugs, new noninvasive coronary screening methods, advanced blood testing and a much more accurate understanding of how heart attacks happen. Although I had been practising a form of what I like to call 'aggressive prevention' for years, it wasn't until the late 1990s that I was able to take advantage of all these new strategies and implement the heart disease prevention programme I use today.

Now, thankfully, I am hard-put to remember the last time I got a late-night call from an Accident and Emergency department telling me that a patient of mine had suffered a heart attack. I don't have 40-, 50-, or 60-year-olds in my practice suffering heart attacks or strokes. And among people whom I've treated over a period of time, I rarely find it necessary to refer them for invasive procedures such as angioplasty or bypass surgery. I don't pick only heart-healthy patients, either. I treat primarily high-risk men and women with multiple risk factors and often a family history of heart disease. In fact, many of my patients have come to me after already suffering a heart attack at a young age. If they follow my programme, they don't go on to have another.

As I've said, this is not just *my* experience. One of the best-kept secrets in medicine today is that many doctors who practise aggressive prevention have essentially stopped seeing heart attacks and strokes among their patients. When we meet at conferences and compare notes, it's common to hear 'I've hardly had a heart attack in my practice this entire year' and 'If hospitals had to rely on my referrals for surgery, they'd have very quiet operating rooms.' We don't wait until our patients are crippled by chest pain or in the throes of a heart attack to act. At that late stage, an invasive approach is usually essential. Instead, we use the latest technology to identify people who are at high risk for a heart attack years before they experience any symptoms. We educate our patients about the right diet and exercise. And we prescribe cholesterol-lowering drugs and other medications that are proven to help prevent heart attacks and strokes.

We closely monitor our patients and our perseverance pays off. They stay healthy, happy and nearly always heart attack free. Watching patients who had a parent or sibling die of heart disease before the age of 50 reach their sixties – and often well beyond – has brought me my greatest satisfaction as a doctor. There is usually nothing routine about saving lives. Yet, in cardiology practices using aggressive prevention techniques, saving lives has become routine. My programme works because it is a synthesis of what I have learned over the years from so many leaders in cardiology research and practice, and I owe them a great debt of gratitude. In the Foreword to this book, I have named those who have had the greatest influence on me.

Millions Are Missing Out

Despite all the advances and our proven success, I am frustrated that more people aren't getting the preventive care enjoyed by my patients and the patients of other preventive doctors. In fact, heart disease is by far the number one killer in the United States, accounting for 1 in 5 deaths annually. Statistics from the UK show that in 2005 heart disease was also the leading cause of death in England and Wales with 1 in 5 men and 1 in 6 women affected. And it's not just the stereotypical middle-aged or older man who falls victim. Heart disease is an equal-opportunity killer – over 113,000 women died of cardiovascular disease in 2004 in the UK. *And women, take note:* if you have a heart attack, you are twice as likely as a man is to die from it. I want you women readers to realize that what I say in this book is as relevant to you as it is to your husband, sons, father and brothers.

Most deaths from heart disease result from a condition known as *atherosclerosis*, or 'hardening' of the arteries, which occurs when artery walls are gradually filled by plaque, a toxic soup consisting mainly of cholesterol, inflammatory cells and scar tissue. But all plaque isn't created equal. A heart attack occurs when a *soft, cholesterol-rich plaque* bursts, resulting in the formation of a blood clot that blocks the flow of blood to the heart. (The mechanism of most strokes is similar, except that it occurs in the arteries in or leading to the brain.)

Despite the fact that most heart attacks are preventable, there are about 865,000 new and recurrent heart attacks each year in the US and about 268,000 in the UK. And notwithstanding what preventive cardiologists are seeing every day, *the total number of invasive heart procedures is actually on the rise in the US.* More than 1 million angioplasties are performed each year to open clogged arteries. In addition, some 467,000 coronary bypass operations are performed annually in the United States. Rates are lower in the UK but still around 28,500 coronary bypass operations and 39,000 angioplasties are carried out annually.

Patients are often told that having angioplasty or bypass surgery will prevent them from having a first or second heart attack. In the majority of cases, this simply is not true. While angioplasty (which involves opening a blockage by inflating a balloon at the end of a catheter) can be lifesaving when performed early in the course of a heart attack or when symptoms are severe, it is too often being done on patients with mild or no symptoms of heart disease. In other words, this invasive procedure is being performed on people who are otherwise leading normal lives and for whom opening a chronically blocked artery will do *nothing* to prevent a future heart attack. And while bypass surgery (which reroutes bloodflow around blockages in the coronary arteries using veins and/or arteries transplanted from other parts of the body) can be lifesaving or life-extending in certain people, too many patients are undergoing this very serious procedure even though it will neither prolong their lives nor make them feel better.

Why Do So Many Doctors Practise Intervention?

So...the question is, if we preventive cardiologists are able to sharply reduce the incidence of heart attacks among our patients, and if we have virtually eliminated the need for invasive procedures such as cardiac surgery, why are hundreds of thousands of people still getting heart attacks, undergoing these procedures, and dying from heart disease? What is it that we are doing that other doctors are not? And more importantly, why aren't they doing it? The answers to these questions speak volumes about the current state of the practice of medicine.

First and foremost, cardiologists who practise aggressive prevention understand that the *real* cause of a heart attack is different from what is commonly believed. When I was in medical school in the 1970s, my classmates and I were taught what I call the 'plumbing model' of heart disease. We learned that a heart attack results from a blockage in a major coronary artery caused by a gradual buildup of plaque, in much the same way that a clogged kitchen sink results from a gradual buildup of sludge in a drainpipe. The theory was that as an artery became more and more clogged with plaque, it would narrow to the point that bloodflow to the heart would be cut off.

About 20 years ago, cardiac researchers began to poke holes in the plumbing model. They had noticed that it was not the largest, so-called obstructive plaques seen on angiograms that caused most heart attacks. Instead, it was smaller plaques within the inner lining of the vessel walls. These plaques are like little pimples, but instead of being filled with pus, they are filled with cholesterol. When these cholesterol pimples pop, they cause tiny injuries to the vessel wall. To begin to heal the injury, a blood clot forms, just as it does when your skin is cut. If the clot is large enough to block an artery, blood does not get to the portion of the heart muscle supplied by that artery, and that part of the heart muscle dies. This is a 'heart attack'; if enough heart muscle is compromised, the heart cannot function, and heart failure or death results. But, as you will learn in Chapter 2, most of these plaque ruptures do not cause a heart attack or any symptoms at all.

So, if a procedure to push back or bypass the blockages isn't the best treatment, what is? How do we deal with these cholesterol-filled soft plaques that can still grow, rupture and cause heart muscle damage? The answer is found in the programme I offer in Part 2, which uses diet, exercise and medications to literally heal the vessel walls and return them to their natural, healthy state. In many ways, we are only as old as our blood vessels. With the proper techniques, I have seen that we can actually make our blood vessels younger.

I like to characterize the growing number of doctors using an aggressive prevention approach to heart disease as the 'healers', in contrast to the 'plumbers', who primarily use an interventional approach. The science and the future belong to the healers, but far too many patients (the great majority, in fact) are being treated according to the plumbing model. For example, it is estimated that only about 50 per cent of high-risk heart patients who would benefit from taking a potentially lifesaving statin drug to lower their cholesterol are being prescribed one – and this is a conservative estimate. The fact that people aren't being treated with the appropriate noninvasive medical therapies, whether that means a statin drug, a blood pressure medication, a heart-healthy diet, an exercise programme, or smoking cessation, helps explain the persistently high rates of angioplasty and bypass surgery. This is costing us dearly from both a human and economic perspective.

It has been the rule rather than the exception that new medical approaches, even those that have solid scientific backing, are slow to be integrated into everyday practice. Today, if surgeons went from patient to patient without washing their hands or sanitizing their instruments, you would be appalled. Yet back in the mid-1800s, this was standard practice, and as a result, nearly half of all surgery patients died from postoperative infection. One would think that when, in the 1870s, renowned British doctor Joseph Lister demonstrated that measures such as hand-washing, sterilizing surgical equipment and cleaning wounds could reduce patient death rates dramatically, his fellow doctors would have readily adopted his lifesaving techniques. In fact, most doctors in his own country refused to believe him. Two decades would pass before aseptic surgery would become standard practice in England. I mention this because, when it comes to the willingness and speed of the medical community to embrace new approaches, things haven't changed all that much.

Breaking the Back of the Health-Care System

There are currently incentives for hospitals to cling to the old way of doing things. Current reimbursement policies of our hospital care system favour the plumbing approach. The funding system is such that most income is generated in specialist heart units by performing procedures rather than by practising prevention. In many cases, this is a holdover from the days when there were few effective preventive strategies for heart disease or, for that matter, many other diseases. As a result, you don't see many hospitals featuring 'preventive care units'. Instead they boast of their 'cardiac care units', designed for the invasive procedures that are vital sources of income. Doctors are being paid to treat disease, not to prevent it.

But consider for a moment the cost of *not* implementing an aggressive programme to prevent heart disease. The fact that we are wasting so much money on treating late-stage heart disease has the potential to break the back (and the bank) of the health-care system now that baby boomers are ageing. Why? Because we are getting fatter and suffering more diabetes than ever before. As I noted earlier, the causal link between diabetes, obesity and heart disease is well known. In addition, some 9 million of us have already reached the age of 65 or older, the stage of life when the risk of heart attacks and strokes is the greatest. And as the baby boomers age, this high-risk population will swell. There is no question that if we do not change things, the already high cost of health care will converge with the increased medical demands of the ageing baby boomers to overwhelm the system.

I am a third-generation doctor. My father was an ophthalmologist, and my grandfather was first a paediatrician and later an ophthalmologist as well. This has given me a long-term perspective on how the economics of health care have hurt the doctor-patient relationship, which is the very thing that attracted many of us to the practice of medicine in the first place. Today, patients feel that their doctors don't listen, often don't care, and are always in a hurry. Doctors feel burdened by the massive amount of paperwork. No wonder it's virtually impossible for many of us to take the time we want with our patients. I believe that the situation is critical, but treatable.

Your Role as a Medical Consumer

Patient education and good communication are essential parts of my practice. I have found that patients who understand the reasons behind my recommendations are much more likely to follow them.

Knowing more about cardiovascular disease is essential if you are going to benefit from the revolution in cardiac care. Because of the constraints on the NHS, you will need to play an active role in preserving your own health. In this book, you'll learn how.

If you have a healthy cardiovascular system, you will learn how to keep it that way for the rest of your life. If you have a family history of heart disease, you will learn how to keep from being a victim of your genes. If you have already suffered a heart attack or stroke or have undergone angioplasty or bypass surgery, you will learn how to dramatically reduce your risk of further events and a premature death.

Heart disease may be the number one killer, but it doesn't have to kill you.

Dr Ted Feldman

'When you are treating people aggressively with cholesterol-lowering medications...you don't get heart attacks. You've cured the disease.'

The first angioplasty was performed in 1977 when I was still in medical school, and I remember thinking, 'This is really cool. We're opening blocked arteries with balloons and little catheters. We can save lives. This is what I want to do.' I became a very proud interventional cardiologist. I judged my entire self-worth as a person and a doctor by how many procedures I did every day. I had a thriving practice, but I only got to see people when the building was burning down. Which is ironic, because my dad was a fire chief in New York City and actually did run into burning buildings. But I also felt like I was spending my days putting out fires of a different sort.

Over time, things changed for me personally and so did the practice of cardiology. In the mid-1980s, my mother was diagnosed with very high cholesterol. Her total cholesterol was more than 7.8 mmol/L and her triglycerides were more than 5.6 mmol/L. I knew that with numbers like that she was at very high risk of developing heart disease. And she probably would have, but she was one of the first patients put on a new experimental drug called a *statin,* which at the time was not widely available in the United States. Once she was on the drug, her numbers went way down. I thought taking the drug made a lot of sense. Trying to prevent plaque from building up seemed to be a better approach than what I was doing every day, which was removing it. It dawned on me that if we could get cholesterol levels low enough at some point, I wouldn't have to perform any procedures. I bought into the 'lower is better' philosophy early on. When I started telling my patients and other doctors this, they thought I was crazy. Now it's the mantra of the day. And, by the way, it worked for my mum. She's in her eighties now, and her heart is fine.

I was too much of a coward to have my numbers checked until 1994, when I was 39. My numbers were bad – really, really bad. My total cholesterol was 7.1 mmol/L, my triglycerides were 6.4 mmol/L, my LDL ('bad') cholesterol was 4.9 mmol/L, and my HDL ('good') cholesterol was 0.7 mmol/L. I wasn't overweight or anything; I'm actually quite fit. But I inherited a genetic condition called type 2 familial heterozygous hypercholesterolaemia from my parents. We all knew that cholesterol was bad, but we didn't have any overwhelming evidence that lowering cholesterol with statin drugs would actually save lives. So I didn't take one. Then the 4S study (the Scandinavian Simvastatin Survival Study) was presented at the American Heart Association's meeting in 1994. It provided clear evidence that the lower your cholesterol numbers are, the better. I immediately went on a statin drug and since then other drugs too, including niacin and ezetimibe (Ezetrol). And I started prescribing statins for my patients. My reasoning was, we now have these great drugs, so why not try to get people's cholesterol down as low as possible?

In 2000, I went in to see Arthur Agatston, a friend of mine, for a heart scan, and I found out that my Calcium Score was in the 75th percentile for my age. This meant that I was at higher risk than 75 per cent of other men my age. I decided to go on the South Beach Diet, not to lose weight – I was 1.83 metres (6 ft) tall and 92 kg (14½ stone) then and still am – but because it's the most heart-healthy diet around. So now I take my medications, I work out, and I follow the South Beach Diet lifestyle.

This approach has worked. My numbers are great. My total cholesterol is 3.4 mmol/L, my LDL is 1.6, my HDL is 1.46, and my triglycerides are 0.58. When I went in for a follow-up heart scan, my condition was stable. I had not developed any new plaque. We had, in effect, stopped the progression of my heart disease in its tracks.

Today, that's exactly what I do in my practice, and it's made a huge difference for my patients. The best illustration I can give is that 20 years ago, I would see about five ST-elevation myocardial infarctions (MIs) a week. That's the most life-threatening type of heart attack you can have. I'm now in a practice with six cardiologists and an active database of 10,000 patients whom we've seen in the past 24 months. We don't see five ST-elevation MIs a year among our outpatients! We don't see them because when you are treating people aggressively with cholesterol-lowering medications and you bring LDL levels down to 2 mmol/L or less for very high risk people and 3 mmol/L or less for those at moderately high risk, you don't get heart attacks. You've cured the disease for the most part. There are still people getting heart attacks and strokes, but those are people who aren't being treated medically.

(continued)

Now that we've been treating people longer and longer with these drugs and moving their cholesterol levels lower and lower, I'm down to doing very few invasive procedures a week – my patients don't need them. Over the past 5 years, only one of my patients has had a heart attack. He was a cop on a bicycle chasing a robbery suspect in Miami, and in the process of apprehending the perpetrator, he had a heart attack and had to have emergency bypass surgery. He's doing fine, but that is literally the only heart attack I've seen in my practice in 5 years.

When I'm asked how my practice has changed, I like to say, 'I've put myself out of the intervention business. I'm in the prevention business.' I do a lot of clinical research, I publish in professional journals, and I've become a major advocate for prevention.

The truth is, lower is better. Our goal is to get cholesterol lower, blood pressure lower, blood sugar lower, and weight lower. As I often say, lower is better except for your bank account and your HDL. ∎

2

WHY 'PERFECTLY HEALTHY' PEOPLE GET HEART ATTACKS

About 25 years ago, when I was codirector of the Noninvasive Cardiology Laboratory at Mount Sinai Medical Center in Miami Beach, Florida, performing heart ultrasounds and exercise stress tests, I got a call from a doctor who told me that one of his patients had just suffered a heart attack. He was puzzled because this patient had recently passed an exercise stress test...administered by me! I was very upset by this news and rechecked the test results to see if I had made any mistakes. After careful review, I couldn't find any errors in my analysis. The stress test was normal, and the patient had shown excellent exercise capacity. I remember feeling very frustrated. We were working with the best technology available, yet it wasn't good enough to detect a heart attack that was only weeks away.

Today, we do have other noninvasive tests that are much better at predicting the likelihood of a future heart attack. A normal stress test does not mean there aren't any potentially lethal soft plaques growing inside the lining of your coronary arteries that could rupture and cause a heart attack at any time. All it means is that the bloodflow to your heart was fine on the day you took the test. Unfortunately, that doesn't mean that the bloodflow will still be fine tomorrow.

Recently, I was at a dinner party when another guest, upon hearing that I was a cardiologist, turned to me and said, 'My friend just passed his annual physical with flying colours. Two days later, he had a heart attack. How could this happen?' I'm sorry to say that I hear stories like this almost as often today as I did 25 years ago. The fact is, back then, we had an excuse. We didn't know any better. Today, we do. We know that someone can look great on paper – pass a standard exercise stress test with flying colours, have good cholesterol scores, and never have had a sick day in his or her life – but still have arteries that are a diseased and potentially lethal mess. Today we have access to cutting-edge diagnostic tests that can identify these high-risk people early enough to prevent them from having heart attacks in the first place.

The problem is that many patients destined for heart problems don't get the benefit of our most accurate tests (including presidents of the United States, as you will see in Chapter 6). Many seemingly perfectly healthy people are 'suddenly' getting heart attacks because their arteries are *not* perfectly healthy and they don't know it. With the proper noninvasive tests, these diseased arteries would have been identified, and the heart attacks wouldn't have happened.

In order for you to understand how our thinking about what causes a heart attack has changed, I will give you a short course in cardiology. Don't worry, it won't hurt a bit, and you'll be an expert in no time.

Your Heart and How It Works

Your heart is not an inanimate pump: it is a living, dynamic community of millions of hardworking cells. The heart serves a vital purpose in the body. Its job is to deliver blood to organs that would die without it. Blood contains oxygen and nutrients necessary for the functioning of every cell in the body, including heart cells.

Everyone's heart beats around 70 times per minute, or 100,000 times per day, or about *2.5 billion* times in the average lifetime. This vital organ is programmed to work automatically for every second of every day for as long as you live, no matter what else you're doing mentally or physically. In other words, your heart never rests.

Your heart is located just about in the centre of your chest and is divided into four chambers: the two smaller upper chambers are known as the *left atrium* and *right atrium* and the two larger lower chambers are the *left ventricle* and *right ventricle*.

Oxygen-poor blood enters the right atrium and is then pumped into the right ventricle and through the pulmonary artery to the lungs, where it is enriched with oxygen (and loses carbon dioxide). The oxygenated blood is then carried to the left atrium via the pulmonary veins, from where it enters the left ventricle, the main pumping chamber of the heart.

It is the thick, powerful muscle of the left ventricle that pumps blood to all the organs of the body via the aorta. From a cardiologist's point of view, it is the left ventricle that is the most important chamber because it is the area of the heart most likely to be affected by a heart attack.

As blood enters the aorta, some is immediately directed to the coronary arteries. As you can see from the illustration on page 18, the left main coronary artery divides into two major coronary arteries – the left circumflex artery (LCx) and the left anterior descending artery (LAD). A third major artery, the right coronary artery (RCA), has its own point of origin from the aorta. All of these arteries have branches, which are also known as coronary arteries. They supply the beating heart muscle with blood and oxygen.

If anything obstructs the flow of blood through one of these arteries for more than 20 to 30 minutes, the heart will likely not receive enough oxygen, and the part of the heart muscle fed by that artery will die. This is what happens when you have a heart attack.

Heart failure occurs when your heart muscle is damaged to the point that your heart can no longer pump sufficient blood to the rest of your organs. When your heart is damaged and can no longer pump efficiently, blood also tends to back up into the lungs, making them heavier, which results in difficulty breathing.

The Persistence of the Plumbing Model

More than a century ago, when pathologists first examined the arteries of heart attack victims, they reported that they were hard and inflexible. They named this condition *arteriosclerosis*, from the Latin for *hardening of the arteries* (today we refer to it as *atherosclerosis*). A closer look revealed that the artery walls were not just stiffer, they were also clogged with a yellowish, waxy substance that early medical investigators called *plaque*, a term that we still use today. Cardiac researchers also correctly noted that most heart attack patients had something else in common: one or more of their coronary arteries was blocked, preventing bloodflow to the heart muscle. But these early investigators went on to make two understandable mistakes. First, they surmised

---

THE CORONARY ARTERIES

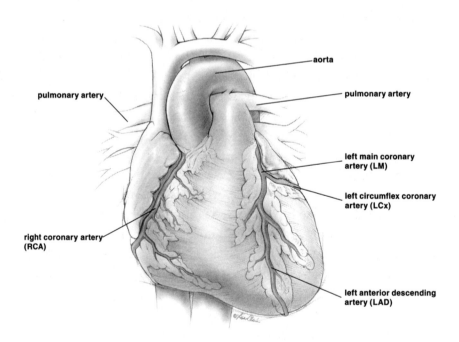

The higher up a blood clot forms when it blocks a coronary artery, the greater the area of heart muscle affected. If the clot occurs in the left main coronary artery, then all of the heart muscle supplied by the left circumflex and left anterior descending arteries will die, causing a deadly heart attack.

that, like gunk in a drainpipe, plaque builds up inside an artery steadily over time, gradually narrowing the opening until it closes, blocking bloodflow. Second, after observing a blood clot at the site of most blockages, they theorized that the clot had formed *after* the plaque had sealed off the artery, causing bloodflow to become stagnant.

In fact they were mistaken. What was actually causing the blockage was not completely understood until fairly recently. Here's what they missed: there are two kinds of plaque – soft plaque and hard (or healed) plaque. It is the soft plaque (the so-called *vulnerable plaque*), which is prone to rupture, that is most dangerous and that most often causes a heart attack. I touched on soft plaque and its dangers in Chapter 1, but I feel it bears repeating here. As I said before, the best way to picture a soft plaque is to think of it as a small 'pimple' protruding from underneath the delicate inner lining of the artery (this lining is called the *endothelium*). The soft plaque is filled primarily with cholesterol. Suddenly, with no warning, the small cholesterol-filled pimple can burst open, puncturing a hole in the endothelium and exposing the contents of the soft plaque to the bloodstream. A blood clot then develops at the site of the 'injury' as part of the healing process. This clot (along with spasm of the affected artery) is what most commonly *causes* obstruction of bloodflow; the clot is not the *result* of obstructed bloodflow, as was previously thought, but is its *cause*!

Why is this point so important? Knowing when and how the blood clot is formed is key to understanding the mechanism of a heart attack, which is fundamental to developing a strategy for preventing and treating heart disease. When the plaque ruptures, causing the formation of a blood clot that compromises bloodflow enough to cause pain, it is called an *acute coronary syndrome* (ACS). If it compromises bloodflow long enough to cause the death of heart muscle, it is classified as a heart attack. As I tell my patients, *if you feel any pain that lasts for several minutes, call your doctor, even if the pain subsides.* You're still at risk. That's because until it heals, the blood clot at the site of vessel injury can still grow and cause a heart attack. This healing process can take several weeks.

The good news is that most plaque ruptures do not result in a heart attack or even in chest pain. In as many as 99 out of 100 ruptures, the clot is largely broken up or dissolved by natural clot-busting enzymes produced by your body. When the ruptured plaque in a vessel wall heals, it scars over (like any cut or wound) and often calcifies. These healed plaques are rarely the source of further problems. They form the hard plaques described earlier.

So why did it take so long for medical scientists to figure out that it's soft plaque, not hard plaque, that is the problem? It's because soft plaque hides inside the artery walls and, on an angiogram, it is often invisible or appears small and nonobstructive.

Why does any of this matter? Using the old plumbing model to design our treatments for heart patients naturally led to an approach that was often counterproductive, because we were treating large hard plaque rather than the real villain, the smaller soft plaque. This resulted in many unnecessary invasive procedures, including surgery. The good news is that now we have a much better understanding of the causes of chest pain and heart attack. We also know how to diagnose heart disease years before it causes symptoms, and consequently we can prevent a heart attack from ever happening.

Chasing the Hard Plaque

So what are the consequences of pursuing a model of heart disease that turned out to be wrong? In the 'plumbing model' of heart disease, the goal of the cardiologist was to clean out the pipes when they became clogged and caused chest pain or shortness of breath, and before they caused a heart attack.

We measured the severity of heart disease by the percentage of the blood vessel that was blocked by plaque. We knew that chest pain did not occur until plaque buildup blocked about 70 per cent of the inside of the artery. We could tell this by the way the heart muscle reacted during strenuous exercise. At high exercise levels, the heart beats faster and stronger. In fact, during strenuous exercise, the heart muscle requires a three- to fivefold increase in bloodflow compared to what it requires to beat at rest. But, when an artery is 70 per cent blocked, it may no longer be able to provide enough blood to the working heart muscle during exercise. This may also happen when the body is exposed to other stressors, including physical or psychological pain.

For example, if you suddenly have to run for a bus or run to return a tennis ball, your heart muscle may require three times its resting bloodflow. If a blockage doesn't allow this increase in bloodflow, then chest pain will result – it's a kind of scream by your beating heart for more blood and oxygen. Shortness of breath, dizziness and other symptoms may also be indicators of inadequate bloodflow to your heart muscle. These symptoms force you to slow down to a pace where the blood needs of your heart can be met, thus preventing damage to your heart due to chronic oxygen deprivation.

Based on the old understanding of heart disease, we believed that once someone's artery was narrowed by 70 per cent, that person was on the way to having a heart attack. It was a foregone conclusion that the obstruction would keep growing until it blocked the entire artery. Chasing the 70 per cent occlusion became the holy grail of cardiology.

As it turned out, we were wrong. A lot of people can walk around with 70 per cent obstructions and have no symptoms. Many people with even more severely blocked arteries don't go on to have heart attacks. Nevertheless, we viewed surgery as the last and only hope for such people.

The False Promise of Invasive Procedures

Since coronary artery disease was viewed as a 'plumbing problem', we became plumbers of sorts, but we used scalpels, balloons and stents instead of plumber's snakes and pipes. We resorted to invasive procedures like bypass surgery and angioplasty to clean out the clogged arteries by bypassing them or squashing what we often didn't realize were almost always healed plaques not destined to cause heart attacks. If a patient had chest pains because of an obstructive 'healed' plaque, then his or her symptoms might be relieved, but the procedure wouldn't prevent a future heart attack. If the person went on to

(continued on page 24)

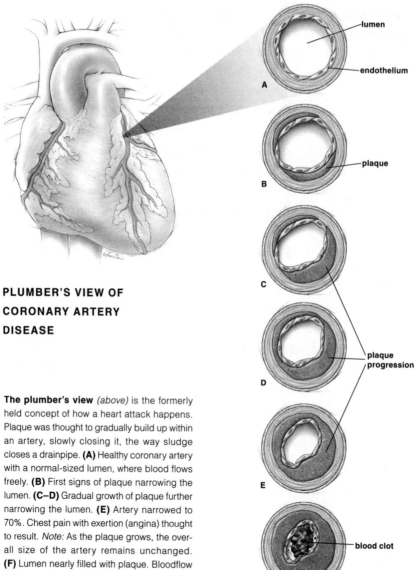

lumem

endothelium

A

plaque

B

C

plaque progression

D

E

blood clot

F

PLUMBER'S VIEW OF CORONARY ARTERY DISEASE

The plumber's view *(above)* is the formerly held concept of how a heart attack happens. Plaque was thought to gradually build up within an artery, slowly closing it, the way sludge closes a drainpipe. **(A)** Healthy coronary artery with a normal-sized lumen, where blood flows freely. **(B)** First signs of plaque narrowing the lumen. **(C–D)** Gradual growth of plaque further narrowing the lumen. **(E)** Artery narrowed to 70%. Chest pain with exertion (angina) thought to result. *Note:* As the plaque grows, the overall size of the artery remains unchanged. **(F)** Lumen nearly filled with plaque. Bloodflow stagnates, a blood clot forms and obstructs flow, and a heart attack results. The belief was that the greater the blockage, the more imminent a heart attack. The logical plumber's approach was to open the artery with angioplasty or to bypass it when partially blocked and before it closed. The plumber's view has turned out to be *all wrong!*

The healer's view *(opposite)* reflects what we now know about how coronary artery disease occurs. **(1)** Healthy coronary artery with a normal-sized lumen. **(2–3)** Gradual buildup of

soft plaque. Unlike in the plumber's view, the plaque grows *outwards* and the artery becomes larger; this is called *remodelling*. Because the size of the lumen is preserved, a large amount of plaque can build up without compromising bloodflow; therefore neither chest pain nor an abnormal stress test result. Without aggressive prevention, **progression to plaque rupture** is likely. **(4A)** Soft plaque ruptures the endothe-

HEALER'S VIEW OF CORONARY ARTERY DISEASE

1
lumen
endothelium

2
soft plaque

3
soft plaque progression

artery begins to remodel

PROGRESSION TO PLAQUE RUPTURE AND HEALING

REGRESSION

4A
platelets
soft plaque
rupture

4B
soft plaque

5A
blood clot
blood clot
injured vessel wall

5B
soft plaque

6A
calcification (hard plaque)
scar tissue

6B
scar tissue

lium. Blood platelets are attracted to the injured site and begin to form a blood clot. **(5A)** The clot extends into the lumen. If it blocks the lumen, then blood can't get to the heart muscle and the muscle dies. This is a heart attack. Administered in time, clot-busting drugs or angioplasty can abort the heart attack. Most plaque ruptures do not cause a heart attack, however. **(6A)** After a plaque ruptures, healing of the injury to the artery wall begins. Scar tissue forms and then calcification, or hard plaque, occurs. Healed hard plaque typically does not cause a heart attack. Hard plaque can be seen on a noninvasive heart scan.

With aggressive prevention, **regression** of soft plaque occurs. Plaque rupture and a heart attack are avoided. **(4B–6B)** Regression and disappearance of soft plaque, leaving a small scar.

experience a heart attack, it invariably came from a soft plaque that had ruptured, one that hadn't been obstructing the vessel or contributing to prior symptoms.

The costs of this plumbing approach have been staggering. But, in our defence, we believed it worked, and we really didn't have good medical therapies until fairly recently. Medications to relieve pain or to lower cholesterol or blood pressure were few, had to be taken several times a day, and had substantial side effects. And they were not very effective compared to today's armamentarium of state-of-the-art drugs. And back then we knew little about the roles of diet and exercise in the prevention or treatment of heart disease. By performing bypass surgery or angioplasty, we felt that we were preventing 70 per cent blockages from progressing to the point of causing a heart attack and death.

If we suspected a problem, we sent our patients for an invasive angiogram, also known as *cardiac catheterization*, a procedure that was and is used to detect and measure artery blockages (see Chapter 8, page 108, for how it is done). Angiography is generally a very safe procedure, but it can have complications of local bleeding, compromised kidney function from the dye that is used (especially in the elderly and in people with diabetes) and, rarely, it can cause a heart attack or stroke.

When I was a young hospital-based cardiologist, our 14-member cardiology group, along with our cardiology fellows (cardiologists in training), would sit together at the end of the day to review the films of the angiograms performed that day. We discussed the films and classified patients into one of three categories. Those who had no disease or who had artery blockage of less than 50 per cent were classified as having 'completely normal coronaries' or 'nonobstructive disease' and were told that everything was fine. Those who had plaque deposits that blocked 50 to 70 per cent of an artery were given a diagnosis of 'borderline disease'. Those who had 70 per cent and greater blockages were considered candidates for angioplasty or bypass surgery. Often, such patients were told that they needed surgery urgently or they risked a heart attack and death. As it turned out, these categories did not accurately reflect the whole story of the patient's risk. We were undoubtedly sending to surgery people who didn't need it and sending home people who had progressive atherosclerosis and were destined for a heart attack. Of course, we didn't know that back then.

The Old Model Didn't Add Up

In the early years of my cardiology training, I was frustrated by a nagging feeling that we weren't doing enough to alter the course of coronary artery disease. These were still the early days of coronary bypass surgery and before angioplasty was introduced in 1977 by Dr Andreas Gruentzig, who was working in Switzerland. I remember asking a cardiology professor of mine whether bypass surgery really worked. He answered that he was confident that he had seen patients survive bypass and live longer than they would have without surgery. This was at a time when most patients who were bypassed had significant symptoms and our preventive medical therapies were almost nonexistent. Studies comparing noninvasive and invasive therapies had not yet been completed. We were treating on the basis of our understanding of coronary disease at that time.

Yet another senior cardiologist I knew back then also shared his opinion on the subject. He noted that there were many post-heart attack retirees living in Florida who had survived for many years with exertional angina (chest pain upon exertion) despite not undergoing bypass surgery. He felt that younger cardiologists did not have an appreciation of the often-slow evolution of coronary artery disease. Upon hearing this, I immediately thought of a fellow with whom I had played doubles tennis occasionally over the previous years. He was in his mid-fifties, and during our matches over several years, he would stop, rest, pop a glyceryl trinitrate (GTN) tablet and then return to the court. I know now that even though he had exertional angina, he did in fact reach retirement and survived many years without bypass surgery.

After I finished my fellowship and practised cardiology for several years, I became aware of a disconnect between what I had learned in my training and what I was observing in the real world. Heart disease didn't behave the way I anticipated it should. For example, we were taught that patients would experience a gradual deterioration in exercise capacity consistent with the gradual narrowing of their arteries. According to this logic, if a patient could walk 20 blocks before feeling pain when his artery was 70 per cent blocked, he would only be able to walk 15 blocks without pain when his artery was 80 per cent blocked, and so on until he could hardly walk a block without feeling pain. Ultimately, the plaque would close off the artery completely and cause a heart attack.

The problem with this model was that it didn't reflect what I was seeing in clinical practice. Patients did not deteriorate slowly over time. Often, no symptoms occurred until their first heart attack. (*Indeed, we now know that roughly half of all people who have a heart attack don't have any prior chest pain at all!*) In those who did exhibit exertional chest pain as their first sign of coronary artery disease, it would typically occur during an unusually stressful activity, such as running up a hill, walking a longer distance than usual (often after a meal), or shovelling snow. The symptoms would not naturally get worse, but rather would require a similarly stressful situation to recur. This is what we classify as *chronic stable angina*.

My tennis partner was such a patient. He would require a glyceryl trinitrate tablet at a similar point of exertion during each match, but at other times he was fine. With examples like this confronting me every day, it seemed obvious that the standard explanation for chest pain being caused by the gradual buildup of plaque in the arteries was just plain wrong.

The Myth of the 70 Per Cent Lesion

There were other pieces of the heart attack/coronary artery disease puzzle that didn't fit. When patients first came to me with chest pain requiring an angiogram, they usually had 70 per cent or greater blockages in more than one artery. Some had complete occlusions – yet they had never suffered a heart attack and had no heart damage. Other patients, who had no substantial plaque buildup, experienced a heart attack as their first symptom! If, as we believed, the clogging of an artery by a large plaque always caused chest pain, then patients should invariably come to the cardiologist when their first artery was 70 per cent blocked. How could a person have no symptoms, feel fine, and pass a stress test one day and then have a heart attack the next? Surely the blockage couldn't grow that fast overnight – or could it? And if angioplasty or bypass surgery eliminated the problems presented by the obstructing plaques, then why was it so hard to show that these procedures prevented future heart attacks? Clearly, we were missing important pieces of the puzzle.

Solving the Mystery

Throughout the 1980s, new and exciting information about the true causes of heart disease began to answer many of these questions. We finally understood that we had been chasing the wrong culprit.

In 1980, a landmark and very courageous study was published in the *New England Journal of Medicine* by Dr M. A. DeWood and his colleagues at the Deaconess Medical Center in Spokane, Washington. It began to change our understanding of what causes a heart attack. Dr DeWood performed coronary angiograms during very early stages of a heart attack. This was gutsy, because a heart attack had been considered a potentially unsafe situation for performing coronary angiography.

What he found was that the earlier the angiogram was performed after a heart attack, the greater the likelihood that there was a complete blockage. In the very early hours after a heart attack, almost all (87 per cent) of the patients had total blockage with a blood clot in the artery supplying the injured heart muscle. When the angiogram was delayed for 12 to 24 hours after the heart attack, significantly fewer patients (65 per cent) had total blockage with a blood clot.

Why was this study so important? It produced strong evidence of what we now know to be true. Heart attacks are most commonly caused by the sudden development of a blood clot that blocks the vessel. Once the clot develops, our body's own defence mechanisms begin to dissolve it, so that when an angiogram is performed hours, days or weeks after a heart attack, we may no longer see a total blockage or even a significant one. Our body is producing anticlotting factors that dissolve the clot. This insight helped us develop the standard treatment for heart attack in the acute stages that we use today – clot-busting drugs to dissolve the clot and angioplasty to squash it or, if need be, bypass surgery to restore circulation to the heart.

Other medical researchers further added to our understanding of heart disease. Thanks primarily to the detective work of pathologists Dr Michael Davies from the United Kingdom, and Dr Erling Falk, PhD, of Denmark, the evidence only mounted that much of what we had believed about heart attacks was wrong.

From the work of these and other medical pioneers, we learned what I suggested earlier – that hard plaque, the primary target of angioplasty and bypass surgery, isn't the culprit we believed it to be. The great majority of heart attacks are caused by the rupture of previously *nonobstructive* soft plaques. But the problem with soft plaques is that you often can't see them on an angiogram, and if you can see them, they are usually less than 70 per cent obstructive. Therefore, we had ignored them.

So what does the hard plaque tell us and is it worth paying attention to? The amount of calcified hard plaque in your arteries provides clues as to whether or not you are likely to have a heart attack. If you have a great deal of calcified plaque, it's a sign that you are experiencing lots of soft plaque ruptures. You've been lucky so far. Your body's natural clot busters have been able to do their job. At some point, however, one of these plaque ruptures may trigger The Big One – the blood clot that eludes your body's natural clot busters and closes off an artery, causing a bona fide heart attack. As you will learn in Step 3 of the South Beach Heart Programme, if you have either a fast CT scan or an EBT heart scan, you will be given your Calcium Score. This score measures the amount of calcified plaque in your coronary arteries and reflects the degree of atherosclerosis that is present. It is a useful tool for predicting who is vulnerable to a heart attack.

Your Heart Performs Its Own Bypass

The new model of heart disease that came out of the research done in the 1980s and 1990s revealed some amazing things about the healing power of the heart. For one thing, it showed why patients who walked around with significant blockages in their arteries could have no symptoms. It turns out that it's primarily because our bodies come equipped with an alternative network of blood vessels that are pressed into service whenever a vital organ such as the heart has an insufficient blood supply. The medical term for this is *collateral circulation*.

Everyone is born with this supplemental network, but the vessels are not fully developed until they are needed. The rest of the time, they function like the spare tyre you carry in your car in case of a puncture. It is currently thought that when bloodflow is restricted, the body produces hormonelike chemicals (more specifically, growth factors) that 'turn on' these dormant vessels, signalling them to inflate and expand. As these vessels become fully formed, they begin to transport blood to the heart muscle, helping to make up for limited bloodflow in the blocked artery. That's why patients can have multiple blockages with normal flow to their heart muscle and therefore no chest pain. If the blockage becomes more severe, more vessels are recruited, and the ones already formed grow larger and carry more blood. *In a sense, the body performs a bypass on itself.*

Many of these natural bypasses are difficult to detect because many of the vessels are so small that they cannot be seen on an angiogram. Only the larger ones show up on an angiogram. Nonetheless, they can transport a significant amount of blood. In fact, in many ways, our natural bypasses are superior to the ones constructed by surgeons. Due to their miniature size, they do not clog up with plaque, even in people who have advanced hardening of the arteries. (Only larger vessels become diseased.) What's more, natural bypasses cost no money, do not require hospitalization, and are free of negative side effects.

From Plumbers to Healers

With our new understanding of the direct role of soft plaque in heart attacks, it's obvious that bypass surgery and angioplasty, when used as a treatment for chronic hard, healed plaque, do not treat the underlying cause of the disease. Although these procedures may relieve symptoms by opening an artery, the sad truth is that even as patients are recuperating from angioplasty and bypass surgery, more dangerous soft plaques continue to accumulate in their arteries and in their bypass grafts.

We now know that the best way to prevent a heart attack is to target that dangerous enemy – the soft plaque. But how do you know if you have plaque in your arteries? Both conventional and advanced blood testing, which I describe in Step 3, pages 204–8, can identify many of the factors that are responsible for the formation of plaque. And having a noninvasive heart scan, which I also describe in that chapter on pages 208–10, can also detect the amount of plaque that's already there. All this good information would be wasted if there were nothing we could do for you or if there were nothing you could do for yourself. But the wonderful news is that with the right combination of lifestyle changes and medications, we can virtually eliminate the soft plaque threat that is the major cause of a heart attack.

3

You May Be at Risk and What You Can Do about It

When I was at school, a friend's father died suddenly of a heart attack. I will never forget how shocked I was that someone who appeared to be so vigorous and healthy one day could be dead the next day. I began to worry about my own father's health. Whenever he was late coming home from work, I was afraid that he, too, had suffered a heart attack. This experience had a profound effect on me and played a role in kindling my interest in heart disease.

Later, as a medical student, I learned that medical science offered little information about heart disease prevention. During my training, I asked a close family friend who was an experienced cardiologist how heart attacks could be prevented. His answer: 'Pick the right parents.'

I was frustrated by his response, but at that time the fact that early heart attacks tended to run in families was pretty much the extent of our knowledge in cardiac prevention. We also knew that men over the age of 50 were more vulnerable than younger men to heart attacks and strokes. And we really didn't think much about women in connection with heart disease, because we mistakenly believed that women were somehow at much less risk for heart attacks! As for prevention, we had virtually no proven strategy for people who had a history of premature heart disease in their families. It was during my training that the results of the earliest studies on risk factors for heart disease began to come to light.

The first evidence that diet and lifestyle could be risk factors for heart disease came from the famous Framingham Heart Study, a long-term look at the lives and health of some 5000 men and women who resided in the small town of Framingham, Massachusetts (see below).

THE FRAMINGHAM HEART STUDY

Whenever I tell my patients to stop smoking or to get more exercise or to lower their LDL ('bad') cholesterol, I owe a debt of gratitude to the Framingham Heart Study. Without it, preventive cardiologists like me would have little advice to give. Before the Framingham study, we knew very little about risk factors for heart disease, and much of what we thought we knew was wrong. For example, we didn't know that high blood pressure put someone at risk of having a heart attack or stroke. Nor did we recognize the role of cholesterol and other blood fats such as triglycerides in promoting heart disease. And until 1960, smoking was not proven to be dangerous.

Launched in 1948, the Framingham Heart Study was the first long-term study of cardiovascular health. It followed approximately 5000 people living in the small town of Framingham, Massachusetts. The first order of business was to conduct a thorough medical examination on all of the participants and interview them about their health habits and family medical history. Did they smoke? What did they eat? How often did they exercise? Did they drink alcohol? Did they have close family members with heart disease?

Following the initial interview, the researchers monitored the health of the volunteer subjects over a period of several decades. This gave the researchers the opportunity to correlate the health of the volunteers with the data they had gathered at the beginning of the study. For example, they would be able to see if smokers had a higher incidence of heart attacks than nonsmokers. They could determine if high blood pressure was more common in people who were overweight. This was plodding, tedious work, but it ultimately produced a great deal of lifesaving information.

The Framingham study made quite an impression on me as a young doctor. I particularly admired Dr William Castelli, who took the reins as director of

---

Commissioned by the US Public Health Service in 1948, this study has produced a wealth of information on risk factors for heart attacks and strokes. Framingham data taught us about the important connection between heart disease and cholesterol as well as between heart

Framingham in 1979 and held that position until 1995. He deserves tremendous credit not just for his research but also for travelling around the US spreading the prevention message in an especially entertaining way. I attended as many of his lectures as I could in the 1980s, and they bolstered my interest in cardiac prevention. His positive message was that it was possible to prevent heart attacks and strokes by improving bad cholesterol numbers through lifestyle changes and medications. We didn't have all the tools back then that we have now, but it was an excellent jump start in the right direction.

The important work of Framingham continues. In 1971, the investigators recruited 5124 children of the original volunteers and their spouses for a second influential study – the Framingham Offspring Study – which is shedding new light on genetic risk factors. Another group of researchers is studying the various subcategories of LDL and HDL cholesterol, deepening our understanding of the genesis of atherosclerosis.

Unfortunately, much of this information has yet to filter down to the public. For example, in a 1997 survey of heart attack victims who had high blood pressure, 85 per cent did not know that hypertension increased the risk of a heart attack. An alarming 26 per cent of the victims who smoked cigarettes did not know that smoking is a major risk factor for heart attacks and strokes. This tells us that tens of millions of people are in the dark about what puts them at risk for cardiovascular disease. They don't know what lifestyle changes they can make to lower their risk, and they may not understand their risk factors well enough to comply with their doctors' recommendations. To obtain more information on the Framingham Heart Study, see Helpful Resources, page 247.

disease and smoking. The Framingham study was also one of the first trials to include women, and it provided some early insight into the differences in the way men and women experience heart disease. It was, in fact, the Framingham study that coined the term *risk factors*.

Today, thanks to information gleaned from the Framingham study and subsequent investigations, we have a better understanding of the factors that cause heart attacks and strokes. I designed the questionnaire in this chapter to help you understand where you stand in terms of your own risk factors. If you are at risk, my prevention approach will enable you to minimize that risk. But there's an important point that I can't stress enough. Obvious risk factors tell only half the story. *Many heart attacks occur in people with few or no conventional risk factors.* This is why I urge even those of you who think that you are not at risk to take advantage of the new, noninvasive medical tests that I describe in Step 3 of the programme. Although many of these would have to be performed privately in the UK, by having these advanced tests, you will have a far more complete picture of your cardiovascular health.

So Where Do You Stand?

How many known risk factors for heart disease do you have? Answering this question is an essential first step in implementing your own aggressive heart disease prevention programme. The questions on pages 36–39 will give you a general idea of your risk level, based on information you are likely to have from your last medical examination and facts you already know about your family history and lifestyle. A copy of your most recent lab test results will help you answer questions about your blood fats (*lipids*), such as cholesterol and triglycerides. If you don't know the answers to some of the questions – for example, your blood pressure or cholesterol levels – you should check with your doctor. If you haven't had a physical examination recently, make an appointment to have one, and be sure to discuss the advanced screening tests that I recommend. In the UK it is recommended that everyone over the age of 40 has screening for lipid and glucose levels.

You will notice that there are two questionnaires, one for men and one for women. We now know that the risk factors for men and women are somewhat different, and the questionnaires reflect this. After you complete the questionnaire, turn to pages 40–59 for a discussion of what your answers mean.

Ben's Story

'I looked at my test numbers and had no idea what they meant.'

I didn't know much about my risk for heart disease. I guess I depended on my doctor to keep me informed, and he didn't tell me enough. And I never knew enough to ask the right questions. The last time I saw him for a checkup, he ordered blood tests. I got a letter in the mail with the results. My cholesterol was 6.3 mmol/L, and there was an arrow pointing up. I guessed that the arrow meant it was too high. My triglycerides (I didn't know what those were) were 1.7. Another upward arrow. My HDL was 1.1. No arrow. Must have been okay. Then there was 'LDL/ HDL' and 'Cholesterol/HDL', followed by some more numbers. That letter was not helpful at all. I looked at my test numbers and had no idea what they meant. All I knew was that something must have been wrong, because he wrote on the sheet: 'Elevated lipids. Strict diet. Recheck 3 months.' Seven words. He also included a sheet about starting the strict diet. I didn't go on the diet. I just handed the information to my wife, and she filed it away. The next time I saw my doctor, he didn't mention anything about the letter, the tests or the diet. It was like the examination never happened. I changed doctors. At least I was smart enough to do that.

Not long after I started seeing my new doctor, I started having mild chest pains. The new doctor gave me a comprehensive battery of tests including a stress test, a heart scan and advanced blood testing for CRP and homocysteine. The difference was that she explained what all the tests were and what the results meant. I'm lucky. Not only did I find a doctor who explained things, but my chest pains turned out to be acid reflux. What I learned is that tests are important and so is having a doctor who communicates effectively. ■

JUST FOR MEN

Are You at Risk for Heart Disease?

1. Have you ever been diagnosed with cardiovascular disease, including a heart attack, angina or stroke, or have you undergone angioplasty or bypass surgery?

☐ Yes   ☐ No

2. Are you 40 years of age or older?

☐ Yes   ☐ No

3. Do you smoke or do you have extensive exposure to secondhand smoke?

☐ Yes   ☐ No

4. Have you been diagnosed with diabetes, prediabetes or metabolic syndrome?

☐ Yes   ☐ No

5. Are you taking medication to treat high blood pressure or is your blood pressure greater than 140/90?

☐ Yes   ☐ No   ☐ Don't Know

6. Do you have a waist circumference of more than 102 cm (40 in)? (If you don't know, use a tape measure to find out.)

☐ Yes   ☐ No

7. Do you have a high Calcium Score?

☐ Yes   ☐ No   ☐ Don't Know

8. Do you have an HDL, or 'good', cholesterol level of less than 1.0 mmol/L?

☐ Yes   ☐ No   ☐ Don't Know

9. Do you have an LDL, or 'bad', cholesterol level of more than 3.4 mmol/L?

☐ Yes   ☐ No   ☐ Don't Know

10. Do you have a family history of early heart disease? (Do you have a brother or father who was diagnosed with heart disease before the age of 55 or a sister or mother who was diagnosed with heart disease before the age of 65?)

☐ Yes ☐ No ☐ Don't Know

11. Are your triglycerides greater than 1.7 mmol/L?

☐ Yes ☐ No ☐ Don't Know

12. Is your fasting blood glucose greater than 5.6 mmol/L?

☐ Yes ☐ No ☐ Don't Know

13. Do you have a homocysteine level of more than 12 μmol/L?

☐ Yes ☐ No ☐ Don't Know

14. Do you have a C-reactive protein (CRP) level of more than 3 mg/L?

☐ Yes ☐ No ☐ Don't Know

15. On average, do you spend less than 2 hours a week exercising at least moderately (for example, brisk walking, golf, active gardening)?

☐ Yes ☐ No

16. Do you eat fish at least twice a week?

☐ Yes ☐ No

17. Do you eat fresh fruits and vegetables and whole grains on a daily basis?

☐ Yes ☐ No

18. Do you make a conscious effort to avoid trans fatty acids in your diet?

☐ Yes ☐ No

Just for Women

Are You at Risk for Heart Disease?

1. Have you ever been diagnosed with cardiovascular disease, including a heart attack, angina or stroke, or have you undergone angioplasty or bypass surgery?

☐ Yes ☐ No

2. Are you 55 years of age or older or are you postmenopausal?

☐ Yes ☐ No

3. Do you smoke or do you have extensive exposure to secondhand smoke?

☐ Yes ☐ No

4. Have you been diagnosed with diabetes, prediabetes or metabolic syndrome?

☐ Yes ☐ No

5. Are you taking medication to treat high blood pressure or is your blood pressure greater than 140/90?

☐ Yes ☐ No ☐ Don't Know

6. Do you have a waist circumference of more than 89 cm (35 in)? (If you don't know, use a tape measure to find out.)

☐ Yes ☐ No

7. Do you have a high Calcium Score?

☐ Yes ☐ No ☐ Don't Know

8. Do you have an HDL, or 'good', cholesterol level of less than 1.3 mmol/L?

☐ Yes ☐ No ☐ Don't Know

9. Do you have an LDL, or 'bad', cholesterol level of more than 3.4 mmol/L?

☐ Yes ☐ No ☐ Don't Know

10. Do you have a family history of early heart disease? (Do you have a brother or father who was diagnosed with heart disease before the age of 55 or a sister or mother who was diagnosed with heart disease before the age of 65?)

☐ Yes ☐ No ☐ Don't Know

11. Are your triglycerides greater than 1.7 mmol/L?

☐ Yes ☐ No ☐ Don't Know

12. Is your fasting blood glucose greater than 5.6 mmol/L?

☐ Yes ☐ No ☐ Don't Know

13. Do you have a homocysteine level of more than 12 μmol/L?

☐ Yes ☐ No ☐ Don't Know

14. Do you have a C-reactive protein (CRP) level of more than 3 mg/L?

☐ Yes ☐ No ☐ Don't Know

15. On average, do you spend less than 2 hours a week exercising at least moderately (for example, brisk walking, golf, active gardening)?

☐ Yes ☐ No

16. Do you eat fish at least twice a week?

☐ Yes ☐ No

17. Do you eat fresh fruits and vegetables and whole grains on a daily basis?

☐ Yes ☐ No

18. Do you make a conscious effort to avoid trans fatty acids in your diet?

☐ Yes ☐ No

Understanding Your Risk Factors

How many times did you tick the 'Yes' box? The more times you answered 'Yes' to questions 1 through to 15, the greater your risk of having a heart attack or stroke. If you answered 'Yes' to questions 16 through to 18, you have reduced your risk of heart attack or stroke. But not all of the questions are equal. The first seven questions relate to particularly strong risk factors, and if you answered 'Yes' to any of those, you need to be especially vigilant about maintaining your heart health. And while you can't change your age, alter your family medical history, or undo your own medical history, there are steps you can take to prevent your risk factors from destroying your future.

You may be surprised by what you have learned about yourself and your risk for heart disease. The important point that I want to make is that whatever your degree of risk, if you follow the South Beach Heart Programme and work with your doctor, you will significantly reduce it. You do not have to experience a heart attack or stroke! They are preventable!

Question 1
Past History of Heart Disease

Here's the bad news: if you have had a heart attack, you have a one in five chance of dying within the next 10 years. Now for the good news: you can improve the odds by taking positive steps to protect your heart. My practice is filled with people who came to me after suffering a heart attack and have not gone on to have another. In fact, by following my preventive approach, they improve their heart health over time.

If you have a history of heart disease, getting advanced diagnostic blood testing (see Step 3) is not optional, it's a necessity. It won't be offered routinely on the NHS but can be arranged privately. It's the only way you will be able to find out whether you have the kind of cholesterol-carrying particles in your blood that are good, bad or really terrible. (The really terrible kind accelerates the accumulation of cholesterol under the protective lining of your artery walls, leading to the buildup of the soft plaque that I described in the last chapter.)

Advanced blood testing is also the only way that you will be able to find out whether you have dangerous amounts of other substances in your blood, such as C-reactive protein, a marker for inflammation that can damage the lining of your arteries. I discuss this substance in the explanation of Question 14.

Depending on what type of offending substances advanced testing detects in your blood, your doctor will determine the type of treatment that will be most effective for healing your artery walls and preventing plaque buildup, plaque rupture and blood clotting – in other words, for preventing future heart attacks. Typically, treatment includes the lifestyle changes and medications that I describe in Part 2 of this book. If you have a history of heart disease, you must be especially conscientious about making these changes if you want to save your heart and your life. Unfortunately, cardiac care units are filled with people who did not follow a prevention strategy.

Question 2

Age and Your Heart

For both men and women, age is a major risk factor for heart disease. The older you are, the more wear and tear there has been on your artery walls, the longer and harder your heart has had to work, and the more time you've had to accumulate arterial plaque. It's not surprising, then, that four out of every five deaths due to heart disease occur in people over the age of 65.

Men, on average, show signs of cardiovascular disease about 10 years earlier than women do, and on average, men are 5 years younger when they have their first heart attack. Because men tend to get heart disease earlier than women, many women believe that they are at low risk for heart disease. They are mistaken.

Women *do* get heart disease, but usually later than men because their female hormones generally offer special protection for the heart while they are premenopausal. However, once a woman reaches menopause, usually in her late forties or early fifties, her oestrogen levels sharply decline and her risk of having a heart attack dramatically increases. And by the age of 65, women are even more likely

WOMEN, HORMONES AND HEART DISEASE

It may appear as though women don't get heart disease because they tend to develop it later in life than men, largely due to the protective effects of natural oestrogen. As long as women are having regular menstrual cycles, they enjoy a significant, although not absolute, level of protection. Naturally produced oestrogen is linked with lower levels of LDL ('bad') cholesterol and triglycerides and higher HDL ('good') cholesterol. When a woman's oestrogen production plummets in her late forties to early fifties, she begins to lose her hormonal advantage.

For decades, experts advised women to take hormone replacement therapy (HRT) to protect their hearts as well as to relieve menopausal symptoms and strengthen their bones. Oestrogen's heart-protective properties looked so promising that nearly half of all postmenopausal female doctors took HRT, a rate higher than that of the general public, according to a 1997 study.

That all changed in 2002, when preliminary results from the Women's Health Initiative, a 15-year research programme, caused a dramatic turnaround in the thinking about HRT. Compared with women who did not take HRT, women who took Prempro, a combination of oestrogen and progestin, had a startling 29 per cent increase in deaths from heart disease, along with a 22 per cent increase in total cardiovascular disease. These results stunned

than men to develop high blood pressure. Notably, a woman who undergoes early menopause is at greater risk for heart disease than her peers who are still menstruating and still cycling oestrogen.

Chronological age alone does not tell the whole story. I want to stress that just because you are in your sixties or seventies doesn't mean that your heart health is deteriorating. Recently, I reviewed the heart scan of a 74-year-old male patient who exercised daily and followed a healthy diet. There was absolutely no calcified plaque in his coronary arteries, which meant that his risk of having a heart attack was extremely low. He may have indeed chosen the right parents, but that still doesn't completely account for his good health. Some credit must go to his heart-healthy lifestyle.

the health community and caused a great deal of confusion in the general public.

But as it turns out, the HRT story is probably far from over. A review and analysis of many of the published HRT studies recently appeared in the *Journal of General Internal Medicine*. The authors pointed out possible explanations for the disparities between the earlier observational HRT studies of women who had chosen, in consultation with their doctors, to be on HRT and the more recent controlled trials. One factor that appears to be important is the timing of when HRT is started. Those women who begin it later appear to be more likely to experience heart attacks than those who begin HRT soon after menopause. In addition, much of the increased risk seems to occur in the first year HRT is started and may be due to an increased tendency to develop blood clots in the first year of HRT use.

I wish I could give women more definitive advice on this subject, but at this time the research is just too inconsistent. Whether beginning HRT earlier after menopause and perhaps at lower dosages is safer is frankly unknown at this time. Therefore, any decision on whether to begin HRT should be made with your doctor after careful review of the potential risks and benefits for your particular situation.

That same day, I reviewed the scan of a 58-year-old woman who was overweight and sedentary. Her arteries were *loaded* with plaque, which put her at much greater risk of having a heart attack than my older male patient. My point is that you can have healthy arteries well into old age if you make the right lifestyle and therapeutic choices and take steps to reduce those risk factors that are within your control.

What is really important is the 'physiologic' age of your arteries. Just as we are impressed by the sharp minds of many elderly people, we have also seen that they can have young arteries despite their advanced years. In many non-Western societies, where food is not overprocessed and exercise is part of everyday life, the arteries of the elderly are clean and heart attacks and strokes are rarities.

JoAnne's Story

'I feel younger now than I did 2 years ago.'

I'm 85 years old, and I have pulmonary hypertension (high blood pressure in the arteries that supply the lungs). It can be very serious. When I went to see Dr Agatston 2 years ago, I wasn't doing well. I couldn't walk across the room without getting out of breath. I was overweight and I felt terrible. He put me on a healthy diet and told me to get some exercise. Thanks to that, I've lost 18 kg (40 lb). I breathe a lot better now and I can do a lot more things. I like to walk, but I'm not a youngster. I go to the gym three times a week to walk on the treadmill and do the bike. I do as much as I can. When I get tired, I stop, but I feel much happier and I look much better. I feel younger now than I did 2 years ago. I used to eat a lot of sugar and a lot of junk. Now I don't eat fried foods, and I don't eat sugar. I don't keep it in my house. If you visit me and you want sugar, you have to bring your own! Now I eat a lot of chicken soup with fresh vegetables. I take care of myself. I do my own shopping and my own cooking. I'm still driving. I never expected to make it to this age. But here I am, thanks to a great lifestyle. ■

Question 3
Smoking

Whenever I hear about a young person falling victim to a heart attack, the first question I ask is 'Did the person smoke?' The answer is very often 'Yes'.

At any age, smoking at least doubles your risk of heart disease. In fact, smoking can trigger a heart attack even if your arteries are nearly perfect. Once you light up, smoking narrows your arteries, raises your blood pressure, increases your risk of irregular heartbeat, and makes your blood sticky and more likely to clot. Smoking also lowers your HDL ('good') cholesterol and increases arterial inflammation. This is a recipe for a heart attack. There is a good reason that cigarettes are called 'coffin nails'.

I am blunt with my patients who smoke. I tell them that as long as they keep lighting up, all prevention bets are off. I warn them that they'll age faster and have the telltale wrinkled skin and dry, lifeless hair that go along with smoking. And I shock them by telling them that I think they'll be lucky if they actually *do* die quickly from a heart attack, because a long and lingering death from emphysema or lung cancer from smoking is far worse.

If you smoke, and particularly if you have other risk factors for heart disease, each time you light a cigarette, you're playing Russian roulette with your heart. For example, a smoker who has high blood pressure and high LDL ('bad') cholesterol has 14 times the normal risk of having cardiovascular disease. A woman who takes birth control pills (which increase the risk of blood clots) and who also smokes has a much greater risk of heart disease than does a woman who takes birth control pills but does not smoke.

By the way, you don't need to smoke cigarettes yourself to experience their negative effects. According to a sobering study published in 2005, simply spending time every day in a smoke-filled environment makes you one-third more susceptible to heart disease than a person who smokes a pack a day. Laws that prohibit smoking in public places may be lifesaving.

The good news is that as soon as you stop smoking, your risk of heart disease begins to decline. According to the US Surgeon General, 20 minutes after you quit smoking, your blood pressure returns to the level it was at before you smoked that last cigarette. Within 2 weeks, your risk of suffering a heart attack begins to decrease. Within 1 to 2 years after you quit smoking, your risk of heart disease nearly returns to normal.

If you want help in your effort to stop smoking, talk with your doctor. Medications, including bupropion (Zyban) and the recently released varenicline (Chantix), have helped several of my patients stop smoking. You can also take advantage of the advice and support offered by various organizations and websites (see page 247 for further information).

Question 4

Diabetes, Prediabetes and Metabolic Syndrome

If you are aged 40 to 70, the odds are around 30 per cent that you answered 'Yes' to the question about whether you've ever been diagnosed with prediabetes, diabetes or metabolic syndrome. Shocked by this statistic? You should be! Not long ago, diabetes and prediabetes were rare. Now they are virtual epidemics putting millions of us at high risk of heart disease. In fact, diabetes is such a strong risk factor for heart disease that medical professionals define it as a 'coronary heart disease risk equivalent'. This means that a person with diabetes has the same high risk of a heart attack as someone who has already had one. Approximately 50 to 70 per cent of people in coronary care units have prediabetes or diabetes. *Women, take note:* if you have diabetes and have suffered a heart attack, you have an even greater risk of having another heart attack or heart failure than a man who has diabetes and has suffered a heart attack.

Diabetes is well known as a disease characterized by the body's inability to process sugars and starches. Less well known are the problems that people with diabetes have processing fats in their diet.

There are two common types of diabetes: juvenile-onset, or what's now known as type 1 diabetes (which usually appears abruptly before the age of 30), and adult-onset, or type 2, diabetes. About 9 out of 10 people with diabetes in the UK have type 2. Prediabetes, sometimes called *metabolic syndrome, insulin resistance* or *Syndrome X*, will lead to full-blown type 2 diabetes if it goes unchecked. The difficulty with processing fats and the risk of heart attack and stroke begin in the prediabetes phase, which is defined as a blood sugar level of 5.6–6.9 mmol/L.

The problem with type 2 diabetes and prediabetes is that people who have these conditions process fats abnormally, leading to low levels of good HDL and elevated levels of triglycerides. They also have more small HDL and more small, dense LDL (see the explanation of Question 9, page 51). In addition, they often have high blood pressure and more inflammation in their arteries, strong risk factors that I'll talk more about in the next chapter.

To help reduce these risks, national guidelines recommend that people with diabetes keep their blood pressure below 130/80. Giving up cigarettes is even more important for people with diabetes than it is for others, because smoking and diabetes are a deadly combination.

Type 2 diabetes is also closely linked with obesity (see Chapter 5), which explains why, as populations in the West get fatter, the rate of type 2 diabetes is soaring. What is even more alarming is that there are millions more 'diabetics in training' today. I am speaking of our children, who, as they grow fatter and less fit, are rapidly becoming prediabetic or even diabetic. Type 2 diabetes can no longer be called an 'adult-onset' disease.

Luckily, type 2 diabetes is largely a 'man-made' disease that we can unmake if we set our minds to it. Exercise, weight loss and strategic dietary changes – particularly eliminating the highly processed 'bad carbs' found in baked goods, breads, snack foods and other starchy and sugary favourites – are all very effective in reversing insulin resistance. I discuss the connection between heart disease and diabetes in more detail in Chapter 5.

Question 5
High Blood Pressure (Hypertension)

High blood pressure, or *hypertension*, is defined as blood pressure of 140/90 or higher, but it isn't as simple as that, as I explain below. The top number measures *systolic pressure*, which is the level of pressure in your blood vessels when the heart beats, pushing blood out into your arteries. The bottom number measures *diastolic pressure*, the pressure in your blood vessels when the heart rests between beats. In the UK, 34 per cent of men and 30 per cent of women have hypertension. That represents one out of three adults, and the number keeps creeping upwards. Up to the age of 45, hypertension is more common among men than women. From ages 45 to 54, the percentage of women is slightly higher, and after that, it is much more common in women than in men. Afro-Caribbeans are at particularly high risk. According to the American Heart Association, the incidence of hypertension in the African American population is higher than for any other population in the world.

Carrying extra pounds, getting too little exercise, and just growing older increase your chance of becoming hypertensive. At least two of these risk factors – weight and exercise – are within your control. But the more risk factors you have, the greater your risk for heart attack.

High blood pressure is dangerous because it stiffens and narrows blood vessels, forcing the heart to work harder. Overworking the heart causes the heart muscle to thicken, like any muscle being worked strenuously. Over time, this can lead to heart failure. Moreover, high blood pressure promotes atherosclerosis by weakening the protective lining of the artery walls and allowing bad cholesterol to burrow in.

As with cholesterol and blood sugar numbers, expert guidelines defining what actually constitutes 'high' versus 'normal' for blood pressure keep changing. The reason for this is that these numbers were originally determined by what the average blood pressure was in the population rather than by what is optimal. The latest numbers are now based on what is considered hypertensive or prehypertensive, but even these new guidelines may continue to change as more information becomes available. As of this writing, blood pressures of anywhere between 120/80 (normal) and 139/89 are labelled *prehypertension. It is also estimated that people with prehypertension may be three times as likely to have a heart attack as those with normal blood pressure.*

Because blood pressure guidelines do keep changing, I prefer to simplify the matter for my patients this way: the higher your blood pressure, the greater the stress on your heart and vessels and the greater your chance of having a heart attack or stroke. The lower your blood pressure, the less the stress on your vessels and the longer you will live.

Rarely are there symptoms of high blood pressure, which is why it is called the 'silent killer'. It is not uncommon for patients to call me in a panic because they took their blood pressure when they had a headache or were not feeling well and found it to be elevated. The real question is 'Which came first, the high blood pressure reading or the headache?' This chicken or egg question is easy to answer. It is the headache or other lousy feeling that came first. In fact, any pain or stressful situation will cause the release of adrenaline and raise your blood pressure. While regular exercise lowers blood pressure, it is normal for your blood pressure to be elevated during and soon after a workout.

Unfortunately, the association of headache and hypertension remains in the popular culture because of a condition called *malignant hypertension*, which today is very rare and seen almost only in those who have had severe high blood pressure that has gone untreated for many years. I did see a rare case of malignant hypertension in an Accident and Emergency (A&E) department setting during my training in the 1970s. But this was in an A&E department that served an economically disadvantaged community that received very little routine medical care. In my practice since then, I do not recall ever seeing a case of malignant hypertension. So remember, blood pressure is an impor-tant issue that must be treated over months and years. It need not be micromanaged.

You can lower your blood pressure by attaining and maintaining a healthy weight, exercising regularly, cutting back on excess salt and eating a diet that focuses on fibre-rich fruits, vegetables and whole grains. I discuss these lifestyle measures in detail in Step 1 and Step 2 of my prevention programme. In addition, your doctor will tell you whether you also need to take a hypertension medication. There are now very effective high blood pressure medications available that have few, if any, side effects. If your doctor recommends that you take one to lower your blood pressure, it would be foolish not to. I explain more about these medications in Step 4.

Question 6
Waist Circumference

Have you found it necessary to loosen your belt a notch or two from time to time? Are you having trouble zipping up your favourite pair of jeans? An expanding waistline is not just a problem for your tailor. The circumference of your waist is an indicator of your odds of having a heart attack or stroke.

If you have an apple-shaped body and carry much of your weight around your middle, you are at greater risk for cardiovascular disease than if you have a pear-shaped body and store fat mainly in your buttocks and thighs or evenly over your entire body. Studies have found that waist circumference is an excellent predictor of who will develop diabetes and heart disease. Belly fat can also make you more vulnerable to a stroke. In a 2005 Israeli study of more than 1000 men, those with large bellies were 1½ times more likely to die from a stroke than men with a more even distribution of fat.

The bottom line is, if you have belly fat, it's very important to get rid of it through diet and exercise. Read more about What Your Waistline Says about Your Heart in Chapter 5.

Question 7
Calcium Score

A Calcium Score is the measurement of the amount of calcium in your coronary arteries, which reflects the total amount of atherosclerotic plaque present. It is an indication of how all your risk factors interact with each other to cause heart disease. The higher your Calcium Score for your age, the greater your risk of a heart attack or stroke. I believe that most men over the age of 40 and most postmenopausal women over the age of 50 should have a heart scan to determine their Calcium Score. A doctor with experience in the interpretation of these scans should review the results and discuss their implications with you. (See Chapter 6 and Step 3 for further discussion of heart scans and Calcium Scores.) *Of all the risk factors discussed here, the Calcium Score is the single strongest indicator of risk for heart disease.*

Question 8
HDL (High-Density Lipoprotein) Cholesterol

HDL is the so-called 'good' type of cholesterol that protects against atherosclerosis by removing cholesterol from the plaque in your arterial walls and transporting it back to the liver, where it is excreted. This is called *reverse cholesterol transport*. If you have an HDL level of less than 1.0 mmol/L for men and 1.3 mmol/L for women, you are at greater risk of having plaque build up in your arteries. Said another way, the lower your HDL, the greater your risk for heart disease; the higher your HDL, the lower your cardiac risk. We often call HDL levels over 2.3 mmol/L the *longevity syndrome* because this amount usually means very low cardiac risk. I instruct such patients to just make sure they drive safely so they will realize their longevity.

I consider your HDL a 'lifestyle factor' because it is influenced a great deal by diet and exercise, as well as by your genetics. One way you can boost your HDL is through good nutrition. Ironically, the low-fat, high-carbohydrate diet that was adopted during the low-fat craze of the early 1980s could actually lower your good cholesterol and increase your risk of having a heart attack. That's because it focused on eating the wrong carbohydrates and eliminating all fats – even the healthy ones. We now know that following the principles of the South Beach Diet, which means eating moderate amounts of good fats and lean protein, as well as plenty of high-fibre, nutrient-dense carbohydrates (like those found in fresh fruits and vegetables and whole grains), can help to raise HDL levels. Even a glass of wine with your dinner may help. I discuss this on page 143.

Another way you can raise your HDL is to stop smoking. A review of 24 studies published in 2003 found an average increase of 0.1 mmol/L for HDL after smoking cessation. This is appreciable.

Moreover, if you are overweight, and especially if you have a predominance of belly fat, you can raise your HDL by shedding some pounds. One good way to do this is to exercise more. Not only does exercising help you lose weight on its own, it will increase your good HDL. The more you exercise, the greater the rise. Marathoners typically have very high HDL levels.

Finally, a number of medications, including niacin, fibrates and to a much lesser degree statins, can also increase your HDL. In fact, niacin is the one drug that can raise your HDL substantially. This action alone is one of the reasons medications can dramatically lower the risk of heart attack. (I'll talk more about niacin and other beneficial medications and supplements in Step 4.)

Question 9

LDL (Low-Density Lipoprotein) Cholesterol

LDL is referred to as 'bad' cholesterol because its particles burrow through the endothelial barrier (the inner artery lining) and deposit cholesterol in the plaques that form underneath the endothelium, in the artery walls. Rupture of these plaques leads to blood clots (and arterial spasm), which can block the arteries leading to your heart or brain and result in a heart attack or stroke. Even though 3.4 mmol/L or higher is a risk factor, ideally, your LDL level should be less than 2.6 mmol/L, especially if you have other risk factors. For patients who have already had heart attacks and for those at high risk, my goal for LDL cholesterol is less than 1.8 mmol/L.

It's not just your overall LDL number that you need to be concerned about, however. *Just as important is the size of your LDL particles.* The smaller and denser your LDL, the greater your chance for heart attack. As you will learn in Chapter 4, advanced blood tests can tell you how many of these harmful particles you have. If your diet is poor – that is, if you are eating high amounts of bad carbs and bad fats – simply switching to the South Beach Diet can help reduce your LDL cholesterol and raise your good HDL cholesterol over time. But in some cases, diet alone may not be sufficient and medication may be required. As I explain in Chapter 7, statin drugs can be very effective in reducing LDL.

Question 10
Family History

Often, my patients who've had one or both parents die of a heart attack at a young age ask me whether the same thing will happen to them. My answer is, 'It doesn't have to.'

The fact that one or both of your parents died prematurely of heart disease does put you at greater risk, but it doesn't make it a fait accompli. There are other factors that will affect your own heart health, including lifestyle. For example, if your father smoked, rarely exercised and ate a diet high in bad carbs and bad fats, his death could have been hastened by any or all of these factors. You may have been dealt a bad set of genes, but there's a great deal you can do to reduce and even eliminate their negative impact. I have numerous patients with bad family histories who still have good hearts, and I have patients with good family histories who come to me with badly diseased hearts.

You may have inherited a specific gene or cluster of genes that makes you more likely to have bad cholesterol and/or other bad blood lipids, which lead to heart problems. In fact, there is a fairly common genetic disorder that results in unusually high levels of the kind of small, dense LDL particles that I mentioned in the explanation of Question 9. There is also a rare genetic abnormality called *familial hypercholesterolaemia,* which affects 1 in 500 people. If you have inherited this mutant bad gene, your total cholesterol may be 9 mmol/L or higher, even if you exercise and eat a heart-healthy diet. Lipoprotein (a) or Lp(a), which I discuss in Chapter 4, also runs in families but is not affected by diet or exercise.

For the treatment of small, dense LDL, getting plenty of exercise and eating a healthy diet is the primary approach. Patients with familial hypercholesterolaemia always require statins along with leading an optimal lifestyle.

Many people know that the cardiovascular health of their parents influences their level of risk, but they are unaware that the health of their siblings matters as well. According to a recent article in the *Journal of the American Medical Association (JAMA)*, if you have a brother or sister with cardiovascular disease, your own risk is increased by as much as 100 per cent. In fact, if you grew up in the same household as your sibling, your sibling's medical history is likely to be even more informative than your parents'. You and your brothers and sisters not only have similar genes, but you also ate similar food and grew up in the same environment.

Question 11
Triglycerides

Triglycerides are the form in which fat is stored in your body's fat cells. Your triglyceride level is almost always strongly influenced by lifestyle. Remember the low-fat, high-refined-carbohydrate diet that I referred to earlier? The one that we used to think was heart protective? It actually elevates your triglycerides. Two decades ago, when I first began putting my patients on this type of diet, which was recommended back then, I was often dismayed to see their triglycerides go up. This, of course, was the opposite of what I was hoping to achieve. We now know that it was not the carbohydrates per se that raised the triglycerides, but the bad carbohydrates – sugars and starches devoid of fibre and other nutrients – that did it.

The same thing happened when I experimented with an extremely low fat diet that was also popular at the time. When I put one patient with a moderately high triglyceride level of 2.5 mmol/L on it to lose weight, he did not lose weight, and his triglycerides soared to over 5.6 mmol/L. His was just one of many cases like this that made me begin to question the conventional dietary wisdom of the time. Today, I recommend a diet that contains lean protein and moderate amounts of good fats (those found in oily fish, olive oil and nuts) and good carbs (those found in vegetables, fruits and whole grains). If patients follow this plan, reductions in triglycerides can be dramatic.

If you have high triglycerides (over 1.7 mmol/L is borderline high) and low HDL (less than 1.0 mmol/L if you're a man and less than 1.3 mmol/L if you're a woman), your risk of heart disease is compounded.

Your triglyceride level can also give you insight into your LDL particle size. In general, the higher your triglycerides and the lower your HDL, the smaller and denser your LDL and the greater your risk of heart disease. If your triglycerides are higher than 2.3 mmol/L and your HDL is lower than 1.2 mmol/L, it is very likely that you have too much small, dense LDL.

There are a number of ways to lower your triglycerides. In addition to eating the healthy diet that I describe in Step 1, losing weight and getting more exercise can help. Medications such as niacin and fibrates are also effective at lowering triglycerides, increasing HDL, and enlarging LDL particle size. You'll learn more about these medications in Step 4.

Question 12
Blood Glucose

For many years, we have known that high blood glucose (sugar) is an indicator of diabetes. Now that we know that people with type 1 or type 2 diabetes and even prediabetes are at increased risk of heart disease, we view high blood sugar as a warning for these conditions.

National guidelines recommend that you keep your fasting glucose level below 7.0 mmol/L. If your glucose level is measured when you have not been fasting, then 11.1 mmol/L is the upper limit. If your level is between 5.6 mmol/L and below 7.0 mmol/L in the fasting state, or between 7.7 and 11.1 mmol/L when you've recently eaten, you meet the criteria for a diagnosis of prediabetes, or insulin resistance. Above these levels, you have actual diabetes and your risk of heart disease goes up even more.

Blood glucose responds to lifestyle changes, including weight loss, exercise and improvements in diet. (For more on diabetes, see Chapter 5.)

Question 13
Elevated Homocysteine

Homocysteine is an amino acid, a building block of protein that if allowed to rise to unhealthy levels in the blood can promote blockage of blood vessels. High levels of homocysteine have been associated with heart attack and stroke, which is why I recommend that people get their homocysteine checked each year. This is not offered routinely on the NHS but is widely available privately. See page 207 for more on this test.

Elevated levels of homocysteine are also associated with depression and Alzheimer's disease. A recent study conducted at Tufts University showed a direct link between high homocysteine levels and the degree of blockage of the carotid arteries, which deliver blood to the brain. And according to numerous studies, mental stress can cause a temporary bump in homocysteine.

For years, we've known that a combination of B vitamins (folic acid, B_6 and B_{12}) can lower homocysteine levels. Therefore, it seemed reasonable and desirable to prescribe this B-vitamin cocktail for people with high homocysteine. In one study, stroke patients were given a vitamin supplement containing these three B vitamins to see if it would lower their homocysteine and help prevent another stroke. The vitamins did lower homocysteine, but they did not reduce the occurrence of another stroke, heart attack, or death. In a separate Scandinavian study, researchers concluded that taking high doses of vitamin B_6 and folic acid in combination may actually increase the risk of heart attacks and strokes. This doesn't mean that you shouldn't get your homocysteine levels down, but I recommend that you do it by consuming *foods* that are rich in vitamin B, and not by taking supplement pills.

In fact, it's possible to get a significant reduction in homocysteine through dietary changes. An article in the *American Journal of Clinical Nutrition* found that those who included specific types of foods in their diets had the lowest levels of homocysteine. These foods included milk, yogurt, peppers and cruciferous vegetables such as broccoli and cauliflower. All of these foods are mainstays of the South Beach Diet (see Step 1), and I urge you to eat more of them whether your homocysteine is high or not.

Question 14
Elevated CRP

C-reactive protein (CRP) is a marker for inflammation. A higher than normal level of this protein circulating in your blood not only increases your risk of having a heart attack, but also puts you at risk for numerous other diseases, from arthritis to cancer. I recommend that everyone have a high-sensitivity CRP (hs-CRP) test (see page 206) as part of the South Beach Heart Programme. Again, this is not routinely offered on the NHS but is easily performed and widely available privately.

Inflammation in the arteries, represented by the level of hs-CRP, is thought to help precipitate plaque rupture. This is followed by blood clotting and vessel spasm, which can lead to a larger clot and possibly a heart attack.

Getting your CRP level as low as possible may reduce your risk of heart attack, stroke and cardiac death. Why is this? New research shows that CRP is associated with reduced nitric oxide levels in the body. Nitric oxide promotes the health of your arteries. A deficiency in nitric oxide can also slow the formation of new blood vessels, which could make your body less efficient at creating a network of vessels to bypass blocked or narrowed arteries (see page 29).

A diet rich in saturated fat and trans fats as well as processed foods can promote inflammation in the body (see 'Inflammation: The Bane of Civilization', page 79). A recent study comparing the health of people aged 55 to 64 years old in the United States to those in Great Britain found that the American subjects had CRP levels that were 20 per cent higher than those of the British. I believe that this difference in CRP is due to the pro-inflammatory fast-food American diet. Adopting the healthy eating principles of the South Beach Diet, which recommends anti-inflammatory good fats as well as other heart-healthy foods, is one way to bring down your CRP.

If you are overweight, losing belly fat can have a dramatic effect on CRP. Fat cells are not passive storage depots; they are 24-hour factories that churn out a host of substances, including chemicals called cytokines, which promote inflammation. In one study, a group of obese women who lost weight reduced their CRP by an average of 26 per cent. People who are very obese and opt for gastric bypass surgery, or *stomach banding*, can cut their CRP level in half. If you are a smoker, giving up the habit will eliminate a major source of inflammation. Exercise is also anti-inflammatory.

Statin drugs and other medications can also help to reduce your CRP level.

Question 15

Sedentary Lifestyle

Our bodies work best when we are physically active, and they break down when we are not. As we age, our sex hormones decrease (even before menopause in women), and we have a tendency to lose muscle and bone. Since muscle and bone require more calories for maintenance than fat does, even at rest, when this deterioration happens, our metabolism slows down, and muscle does, in a sense, turn into fat. To prevent bone and muscle loss and to maintain your metabolism, exercise becomes even more important as you get older.

When you have a sedentary lifestyle, a number of undesirable changes can follow. Your blood pressure goes up, your triglycerides increase, your level of good HDL falls, and you are more likely to gain weight, especially around your middle. This is a picture of a heart attack in the making. Currently only 31 per cent of men and 24 per cent of women in the UK get enough exercise. The solution, of course, is to get up and move. You'll be reading a lot more about how exercise can help your heart in the South Beach Heart Workout, Step 2 of the programme, beginning on page 166.

Question 16
Two Fish Meals a Week

If you're not eating at least two fish meals a week, you are missing out on the heart-healthy 'good fats' that are plentiful in certain types of seafood, especially in oily, deepwater fish such as tuna, rainbow and lake trout, salmon, herring and sardines. The medical literature continues to feature excellent studies on the many health benefits of adding good fats to our diet. According to the American Heart Association, consumption of omega-3 fatty acids (found in the fish mentioned above) can decrease the risk of abnormal heart rhythms (arrhythmias) and even slightly lower blood pressure. As I explain on pages 234–36, omega-3 fish oil supplements are a good substitute for fish. Certain fish are high in mercury and other contaminants and should be avoided.

Question 17
Fresh Fruits, Vegetables and Whole Grains Every Day

What's on your plate at a typical meal? It should be filled with lots of 'good carbs' – fresh fruits and vegetables and whole, unprocessed grains. Unlike highly processed refined carbs, good carbs contain fibre that slows down their digestion, preventing sudden swings in blood sugar that can lead to cravings.

Another benefit of 'good carbs' is that they are sources of thousands of phytochemicals, compounds such as flavonoids and isoflavones that are believed to help protect us from many diseases of civilization, including heart disease. In fact, a recent study linked eating whole-grain foods (such as rolled oats, bran flakes and wholemeal bread and pasta) with a 36 per cent lower risk of coronary heart disease.

To date, there is no pill or capsule that has been shown to duplicate the benefits of whole foods. If you want to take advantage of nature's full bounty, you have to eat the real thing. In Step 1 of my programme, you'll get a lot more information on how adopting good nutritional principles can improve the health of your heart.

Question 18
Avoid Trans Fats

If you aren't already making a conscious effort to avoid eating foods that contain trans fats (aka *trans fatty acids*), you should be. Trans fats are man-made fats found in margarines, shortening, deep-fried foods (including french fries), and any products that contain partially hydrogenated or hydrogenated oil. Refined, processed carbohydrates, including many commercially baked breads, biscuits, crisps, crackers and other snack foods, may contain trans fats. There is no healthy level of trans fats. The more you eat, the worse they are for you. My best advice is, try to avoid foods containing trans fats altogether.

4

What Size Is
Your Cholesterol?

You may think that the title of this chapter is a mistake and that I meant to say, 'What *Number* Is Your Cholesterol?' But the fact is that I really am just as interested in the *size* of your cholesterol as I am in the total number. If that surprises you, there is a good chance that much of what you *think* you know about cholesterol is wrong and that what you *don't* know about cholesterol could be killing you.

Many of you are probably thinking, 'Not again. You're not going to tell us that another time-honoured belief about medicine has bitten the dust.' I know from my patients that the public often thinks that the medical community is conspiring to keep them confused about medical facts. It doesn't help that every new advance seems to contradict earlier conventional knowledge. This feeling is understandable, but I promise you that there is no conspiracy to keep you off balance concerning medical knowledge. It is just that medical knowledge is advancing rapidly. This is good news, because as it advances, we are continuously improving our ability to prevent and treat coronary artery disease.

For example, in the area of advanced blood testing for cholesterol, there has been continuing improvement in our ability to characterize the many types of particles that carry cholesterol and other fats through our bloodstream. This knowledge is extremely helpful in deciding how to design a treatment strategy to slow and even to reverse the atherosclerotic process. But it can be confusing if it is not put in the proper context.

One of the early lessons we learned from the Framingham Heart Study (see pages 32–33) was that total cholesterol is a predictor of heart attacks. What we later learned from the Framingham study was that while total cholesterol is a predictor of future heart attacks, it is not a very good one. In fact, there wasn't much of a difference in the cholesterol levels of those who were destined for heart attacks and those who remained free of heart disease. I was amazed when I first heard the statistic that more heart attacks occur in people with total cholesterol levels of under 5.2 mmol/L than with cholesterol levels of over 7.8 mmol/L.

Breaking the cholesterol down into the bad LDL particles and tri-glycerides and the good HDL particles helped to explain some of the discrepancies, but a lot remained unexplained. Now, with more advanced testing of the various particles that make up a person's total cholesterol, we have a much better understanding of the reasons for the limitations of total cholesterol measurements.

In the late 1980s, when I first began performing heart scans and complete lipid profiles (what I refer to in this book as a *Standard Lipid Profile*), I noticed that the conventional cholesterol profile, including total cholesterol, LDL, HDL and triglycerides, often did not explain what I was seeing on the heart scans and in my clinical practice. Some people whose heart scans produced low Calcium Scores – indicating nearly plaque-free arteries – had fairly high cholesterol levels. This discrepancy didn't make much sense to me or to other doctors and may be one of the reasons why so many doctors were slow to embrace the belief that high cholesterol should be treated aggressively. On the other hand, other patients of mine who had dangerously high Cal-cium Scores – a sign that their arteries were laden with plaque – had low total cholesterol levels. Paradoxically, this latter group often had low levels of bad LDL cholesterol as well. Their total cholesterol num-bers said that their arteries should be in great shape, but their heart scans told a completely different story – that they were in the highest risk category for heart disease.

More to the Cholesterol Story Than We Thought

The lesson that I learned, and that I want you to learn, is that heart scans don't lie. There is a great deal more to the cholesterol story than we knew back then. We now understand that total cholesterol – including your total good HDL cholesterol and bad LDL cholesterol – is just a piece of a larger risk-factor puzzle. We also now understand that there are different subclasses of both HDL and LDL cholesterol that are categorized by size. And that size matters, as I explain on page 64.

The good news is that although the worst cholesterol subtypes can slip past standard cholesterol tests, they are picked up by the more advanced blood tests available today (available mainly through specialist clinics and laboratories in the UK). This means that we can identify people who have this form of dangerous cholesterol early enough to treat them and save their lives. That's why I advise advanced cholesterol testing and that's why, when it comes to cholesterol, you need to know the difference between the good, the bad and the ugly.

The Lowdown on Cholesterol

You may wonder why, if cholesterol is so bad for you, it is present in your body in the first place. The answer is that cholesterol is not all bad and is, in fact, necessary for life. Your liver manufactures cholesterol for a reason: it is essential for the production of cell membranes and sex hormones, such as oestrogen and testosterone. Cholesterol is even added to infant formula because it's necessary for normal growth and development.

We also obtain cholesterol from animal food sources, such as dairy and meat. (Plant foods like fruits, vegetables and pulses contain no cholesterol.) Although cholesterol is essential to life, we don't need very much of it to keep our bodies running well. Our cells take whatever cholesterol is necessary for maintenance and cell repair and store the excess for future use. The problem is that many of us eat a diet that is too high in saturated fat and trans fats, and this can stimulate the liver to produce more cholesterol than the body needs.

As I mentioned earlier, the connection between high total cholesterol and heart disease was made in 1961 by the Framingham study. Back then, we didn't have the technology to distinguish between different types of cholesterol particles. That gradually changed, and by 1977 the Framingham study had established a link between an increased risk of heart attack and elevated levels of LDL cholesterol.

It was also at this time that we began to confuse the public with measures of different cholesterol particles and terms like 'good' and 'bad' cholesterol. During a discussion with a patient recently, she asked me, 'What's the difference between good and bad cholesterol? Isn't it all the same when it's building up in my arteries?' The answer is that it's not the cholesterol itself that is good or bad, but the particles that carry it. These particles are called *lipoproteins* (the *lipo* is short for *lipid*, which means *fat*). High-density lipoprotein (HDL) and low-density lipoprotein (LDL) are two of them. It's the protein part of the lipoprotein particle that acts like a shuttle bus, transporting the cholesterol (and other fats like triglycerides) through your bloodstream to where they are used, stored or excreted by the body. Lipoproteins are necessary for transporting fats because fat is not soluble in water or in blood.

As it turns out, it's LDL, the so-called 'bad' cholesterol, that is doing a lot of the shuttle bus driving. You'd think that this job would make LDL 'good'. But what makes LDL 'bad' is that in excess it can cause us trouble. All cells have special receptors, or binders, that latch onto LDL, pulling it into the cells, where it is used as needed. When these cells have had their fill of cholesterol, they stop making receptors, which allows the rest of the LDL to stay in the bloodstream. Some of this excess LDL deposits its cholesterol 'baggage' in our artery walls – including those of the heart – resulting in the formation of soft atherosclerotic plaques.

The job of clearing the blood vessels of this excess LDL falls to the HDL particles, which is why HDL is often referred to as 'good' cholesterol. The makeup of the cholesterol itself in both LDL and HDL particles is the same; it is the direction in which the lipoprotein shuttle bus is driving that determines whether the particle is considered good or bad. HDL is good because it serves as a scavenger, removing LDL cholesterol from the cells and plaques and carrying it back to the liver for excretion in the bile, which empties into the intestine so it can be flushed out of our bodies in our stool. This is called *reverse cholesterol transport*.

HOW MUCH CHOLESTEROL IS TOO MUCH?

The Standard Lipid Profile, the heart disease screening lab test used by most doctors, measures your total cholesterol, HDL ('good') cholesterol, LDL ('bad') cholesterol and triglycerides. In the mid-1980s, the US government and the American Heart Association joined forces to create the National Cholesterol Education Program (NCEP) to educate the public about the importance of maintaining normal cholesterol. Based on the NCEP guidelines, total cholesterol should be 200 mg/dL or 5.2 mmol/L or less for everyone.

What follows are the NCEP guidelines for LDL, HDL and triglycerides.

THE US NCEP GUIDELINES FOR LDL CHOLESTEROL

99 mg/dL (2.6 mmol/L) or below is optimal.

100–129 mg/dL (2.6–3.4 mmol/L) is slightly higher than optimal.

130–159 mg/dL (3.4–4.1 mmol/L) is borderline high.

160–189 mg/dL (4.1–4.9 mmol/L) is high.

Anything over 190 mg/dL (4.9 mmol/L) is very high.

I advise my high-risk patients to get their LDL down to 70 mg/dL (1.8 mmol/L). There is some evidence, however, that very high-risk people should get their LDL down even lower. *Regardless of risk factors, I think it's advisable for everyone to keep their LDL as low as possible.*

Size Matters

The information provided by the Standard Lipid Profile, which I cover on pages 201–3, is important and offers the first clue as to whether or not you are at risk for a heart attack or stroke. But there is much more you need to know about your cholesterol before you can determine your true risk level or what treatment strategy is best for you. The full story is revealed only when you have more detailed information about your cholesterol metabolism.

My knowledge of cholesterol was greatly expanded when I began to read papers and hear lectures by Dr Robert Superko, an outstanding medical researcher and educator who pioneered advanced blood

THE US NCEP GUIDELINES FOR HDL CHOLESTEROL

For both sexes, optimal levels of HDL are 60 mg/dL (1.55 mmol/L) and over.

While the NCEP Guidelines do not differentiate HDL levels for men and women, the American Heart Association does, and I agree. It defines an HDL of less than 50 mg/dL (1.3 mmol/L) as a risk factor for women and an HDL of less than 40 mg/dL (1.0 mmol/L) as a risk factor for men.

THE US NCEP GUIDELINES FOR TRIGLYCERIDES

149 mg/dL (1.7 mmol/L) or under is normal.

150–199 mg/dL (1.7–2.3 mmol/L) is borderline high.

200–499 mg/dL (2.3–5.6 mmol/L) is high.

500 mg/dL (above 5.6 mmol/L) is very high.

UK GUIDELINES

Joint British Societies guidelines suggest that everyone's total cholesterol should be below 5 mmol/L and below 4 mmol/L for those at higher risk.

Ideally, LDL cholesterol should be below 3 mmol/L and below 2 mmol/L for those at higher risk.

There are no specific treatment goals for HDL cholesterol and triglycerides in the UK/EU but triglycerides above 1.7 mmol/L and HDL below 1.0 mmol/L for men and 1.3 mmol/L for women are used to identify those with increased risk.

testing to predict and to prevent heart attacks. It was from Dr Superko that I learned that the *size* of LDL and HDL particles is as important as – and possibly more important than – the total amounts of LDL and HDL cholesterol. I touched on this earlier, but in order to really understand why size matters, you need to know a bit more about how cholesterol can harm an artery.

Let's begin by taking a microscopic look at our coronary artery walls, where all the mayhem takes place. The inner lining of the walls is composed of a thin layer of cells called the *endothelium*. The endothelium normally provides a tight barrier that keeps most cholesterol from entering the walls. But when the endothelium is injured by elevated cholesterol, inflammation, high blood pressure, smoking or other factors, the barrier becomes damaged and therefore more porous. It's then that the LDL particles can pass through more easily and deposit the cholesterol they're carrying in the artery walls, where it forms plaque. The more damage the endothelium suffers over time, the more porous it becomes. As the artery walls become more porous, more cholesterol enters. The more cholesterol that enters the artery walls, the larger the plaques grow and the more likely they are to rupture. When a plaque ruptures, it leaves a defect in the vessel lining that stimulates blood clotting and coronary artery spasm, the immediate precursors to heart attacks and strokes. This is why protecting our artery linings from injury by reducing cholesterol through diet, exercise and medications is a major goal of aggressive prevention.

Whether and how fast LDL particles breach the endothelial barrier depend not only on the health of the barrier, but also on the number and size of LDL particles. The more particles there are circulating in the bloodstream, the greater the likelihood that more will enter the vessel walls. Smaller, more densely packed particles move through the endothelium more efficiently, depositing more cholesterol and creating more plaques. *Therefore, the number and size of LDL particles taken together is more important than the total amount of cholesterol carried by the LDL.*

One of the problems with the Standard Lipid Profile is that it only tells you your total LDL and HDL and not whether you have many small and dense LDL particles or small HDL particles. This can be misleading because your lipid profile may show that you have a total cholesterol of less than 5 mmol/L and a total LDL cholesterol of around 2.6 mmol/L, which looks pretty good at first glance. But if the cholesterol is packaged in small particles, you could still be at high risk for a heart attack. I discuss this in more detail on the next few pages.

You need to have an advanced blood test to tell for sure whether you have high amounts of small, dense LDL and/or HDL, but one important indication is a high triglyceride level (more than 1.7 mmol/ L) associated with a low level of HDL. You can get both of these numbers from the Standard Lipid Profile.

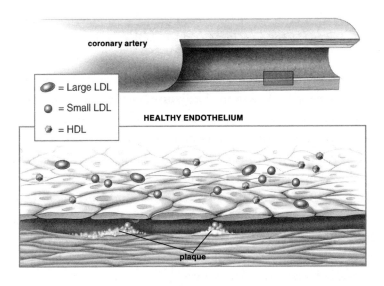

HEALTHY ENDOTHELIUM

= Large LDL

= Small LDL

= HDL

coronary artery

plaque

DAMAGED ENDOTHELIUM

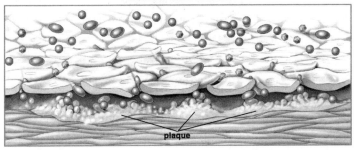

plaque

Top: The endothelium is the inner cell lining of an artery. *Centre:* A healthy endothelium acts as an effective barrier to the penetration of bad LDL cholesterol particles. *Bottom:* When the endothelium is damaged by cardiac risk factors, such as hypertension, obesity, diabetes (or prediabetes) or smoking, it is made more porous to LDL, and there is a greater buildup of cholesterol-filled plaque. Small LDL particles penetrate more easily than large ones do. Good HDL cholesterol particles carry cholesterol from the plaque back to the liver, where it is excreted.

Too Small for the Job

As I noted previously, size matters when it comes to good HDL as well. Not all HDL is 'good' enough to do its job efficiently. Some types of HDL are simply too small. Like shuttle buses with too few seats, small HDL particles, even if you have a lot of them, cannot transport enough cholesterol out of your artery walls. On the other hand, if you have larger HDL particles in your blood, it's a sign that cholesterol is being successfully transported back to your liver for excretion.

When I learned that these small HDL and LDL cholesterol particles are commonly found in patients with type 2 diabetes and prediabetes, it was a real revelation. It explained why so many patients I saw, especially those with diabetes, had high Calcium Scores and established coronary artery disease even though their total cholesterol was below 5 mmol/L.

So why do some people have an unhealthier mix of cholesterol than others? Heredity certainly plays a major role. If you have parents or siblings who had cardiovascular disease at an early age, you are likely to have more of the artery-clogging types of cholesterol. However, eating the wrong foods and being sedentary can also give you unhealthy cholesterol patterns, especially if you have prediabetes.

So what can you do if you find out that you have high levels of small, dense LDL; high levels of small, dense HDL; or both? Losing weight, getting regular exercise, and taking the right medications can increase the size of your LDL and HDL particles. In addition, taking a prescription version of the B-vitamin niacin, which I describe in Step 4, can be very effective. I urge you to talk with your doctor about what's best for you.

The Widowmaker

Beyond finding out the size of your HDL and LDL, there is another reason why you should get advanced blood testing. It's to determine whether you've got high levels of a unique LDL particle known as *lipoprotein (a)*, or *Lp little a* or *Lp(a)* for short. (The lowercase *a* stands for a protein attached to the LDL particle.)

This little particle is a real villain in the cholesterol story, especially in combination with other risk factors, such as elevated LDL. I like to describe Lp(a) as a 'facilitator', encouraging LDL particles to burrow into coronary artery walls. The presence of Lp(a), like the presence of the small LDL particles themselves, also helps to explain the plaque buildup seen in heart scans of people who have seemingly normal cholesterol levels.

Lp(a) has been called the *widowmaker* or *heart-attack lipoprotein* because it is so closely linked with heart attack and stroke. A normal Lp(a) is 30 mg/dL (or 300 mg/L) or less. Researchers have determined that having an Lp(a) of greater than 30 gives you the same risk for heart disease as having total cholesterol of more than 6.2 mmol/L or total HDL of less than 0.9 mmol/L. Lp(a) is especially worrisome because it can increase the risk of heart disease in relatively young people.

Unfortunately, the amount of Lp(a) in your blood is genetically determined. It is a unique lipoprotein in that it is unaffected by the lifestyle measures that improve the other lipoprotein levels. If one of your parents has high Lp(a), you and any siblings have a 50 per cent chance of inheriting it. *And here's something to think about: people who have no known risk factors for cardiovascular disease other than high Lp(a) can still have a 20 per cent higher than normal risk of having a heart attack.*

One of my patients, a security guard, is a perfect example of someone whose numbers hid his illness. When Harry first came to see me, he had advanced heart disease and had already undergone angioplasty and bypass surgery. When I looked at the results of his Standard Lipid Profile, I saw nothing that could account for the alarming condition of his arteries. He had normal triglycerides, and his total cholesterol was an enviable 4.65 mmol/L, with a third of the total being good HDL. I ordered advanced blood work to look for an explanation. When I got the results, I saw that Harry had unusually high levels of Lp(a). This, along with other yet to be discovered risk factors, was the most likely reason for his advanced disease.

As I mentioned, diet and exercise have no effect on Lp(a). I often see high levels in people who are lean, fit and eat very well. The miracle statin drugs do not lower Lp(a), either. Niacin is the only medication that has been shown to significantly decrease Lp(a) levels, and fairly high doses are usually required.

To spare your arteries, it's important that you begin treatment as early as possible if you have high Lp(a). This is one of the reasons that I believe it is critical for people with a family history of heart disease to have advanced blood testing and a heart scan early on.

A Patient Learns a Lesson

Another one of my patients, a policeman named Patrick, learned the hard way how important Lp(a) can be even to people who seem to be the picture of health. Having lost his father to heart disease at a young age, Patrick dedicated himself to eating well and working out. When he came to see me at the age of 54, he was experiencing chest pain with little exertion. This limited my treatment options. When someone has this kind of pain, I switch to an aggressive intervention mode. I immediately sent Patrick to the hospital for an angiogram, and it was a good thing I did. He had a blockage in his left main coronary artery, which is an uncommon situation where coronary bypass surgery is clearly indicated rather than angioplasty or preventive medical therapy. In fact, Patrick did have the bypass.

While it obviously had taken many years for Patrick to develop his extensive coronary disease, he never had any idea of the damage that was being done to his artery walls. Neither did his doctor. Patrick's total cholesterol level and other risk factors were within the normal ranges, so he and his doctor believed he was fine.

Advanced blood testing later showed that Patrick had elevated Lp(a), the one risk factor not affected by his healthy lifestyle. To make matters worse, his HDL particles were also on the small side. When I gave Patrick a heart scan, his Calcium Score was more than 1000, which put him in the highest category of risk for a heart attack. As I've mentioned before, a high Calcium Score means that a person is prone to numerous soft plaque ruptures that could ultimately cause a major heart attack. Just because Patrick had bypass surgery didn't mean he wasn't still at risk.

If Patrick had been given advanced blood testing and a heart scan 5 or 10 years earlier, it would have shown what was developing. We would have known that plaque was building up and that his Lp(a) was elevated. While I am confident that his diet and exercise programme slowed his plaque buildup, it clearly didn't stop it.

Now, finally, Patrick is taking prescription niacin to lower his Lp(a) as well as a statin to further lower his LDL cholesterol as extra protection against his bad genes. My goal is to make sure that he never has to return to the operating table. As long as he keeps taking his medication and continues his healthy habits, I think he'll be fine.

5

What Your Waistline Says about Your Heart

There is an important medical condition so obvious that I can diagnose it without performing a single diagnostic test. I can spot it the instant a patient walks into my office. It's so common that I see it everywhere – at shopping centres, in restaurants, on the golf course, and strolling down the street. It has reached epidemic proportions in the West, particularly in the United States. I'm sure you've seen it, too, among your family and friends, and maybe when you look in the mirror.

The ailment has many names, including *metabolic syndrome, insulin resistance, Syndrome X* and the name I will use, *prediabetes*. Why is it so easy to diagnose? There's one clue that's a dead giveaway: it's your waistline. One of my colleagues says that when a patient's belly is the first body part to enter his office, the diagnosis is made. If you have gained weight in middle age and most of it is in your belly, you are likely part of the epidemic of prediabetes. And if you don't start eating better and exercising, full-blown diabetes will almost certainly be in your future.

Why would a cardiologist be so concerned with your waistline? The reason has less to do with how you look on the *outside* than it does with how you look on the *inside*. I'm worried about what prediabetes and diabetes are doing to your arteries. Both conditions can injure the lining of your vessels and accelerate the production of plaque, greatly increasing your risk of having a heart attack or stroke.

The Belly Fat/Diabetes/Heart Disease Connection

Most people think of diabetes as a disease associated with high blood sugar (glucose) levels. Although this is true, it's only part of the story. In reality, diabetes has as much to do with the way the body handles fat as it does with the way it handles sugar. In fact, long before you become diabetic, when you are still in the prediabetic stage, you are already experiencing harmful changes in blood fats. Too many of my patients minimize my warnings that they are at risk for future diabetes – and heart attack – because they think they have plenty of time to change their ways. But they are wrong – dead wrong. Heart attacks, strokes and death frequently occur in the *pre*diabetes phase. If all this is new to you, it's because the diabetes–fat connection wasn't understood until fairly recently. But it's a very important and often neglected part of the diabetes story.

If you don't know much about diabetes, let me quickly bring you up to speed. As discussed in Chapter 3, there are two major types of diabetes: type 1 and type 2. Type 1 occurs when the pancreas has sustained some type of injury (possibly from an infection) and doesn't make enough insulin. This is the hormone that is responsible for moving the blood sugar and fatty acids (the basic component of fats) that we get from food out of the bloodstream and into the body's cells, where they are used for energy or stored as body fat. Type 1 diabetes typically develops in childhood; it can be treated with insulin injections. Type 2 diabetes, the most common form of diabetes in the Western world today, is another story. Here the body produces enough insulin, but the cells can't use it properly. This condition is called *insulin resistance*, and in those who have it, elevated levels of sugar and fat remain in the bloodstream for longer than normal after a meal, eventually causing serious health problems.

Insulin resistance is a key factor in type 2 diabetes, and it is important to understand how it affects the body. After eating, when your blood sugar rises, insulin is secreted by the pancreas into the bloodstream and then carried into your tissues. There, it locks onto receptors on the cells and facilitates the entry of blood sugar and fat into those cells. As this is happening, your blood sugar gradually drops. That's why it normally takes many hours after a meal for your blood sugar to drop enough to stimulate your hunger for another meal.

This orderly process unravels when you develop that spare tyre around your waist. The more fat you store around your middle, the bigger the belly fat cells become. The problem is, insulin does not attach to swollen fat cells as efficiently after a meal. More insulin has to be produced by the pancreas to overcome the 'insulin resistance' of these larger cells so that sugar and fat can be cleared from your bloodstream.

Our blood sugar levels rise more when there is insulin resistance and more insulin is secreted. Once the extra insulin kicks in, the blood sugar falls abruptly. This rapid blood sugar fall is called *reactive hypoglycaemia*, and it occurs sooner after a meal than the normal gradual fall in blood sugar. This exaggerated swing in blood sugar results in hunger and severe food cravings.

What about the fats floating around in the bloodstream? Remember that after a meal, it is the job of insulin to help transport fats as well as sugar from the blood into the tissues. As you develop insulin resistance, fats accumulate in your bloodstream and hang around much longer than usual. During this time, changes in your blood fats occur – your LDL particles and your HDL particles become smaller and your total HDL is reduced. These changes favour the movement of cholesterol from your bloodstream into your artery walls. As we discussed in Chapter 4, the smaller and denser the LDLs are, the more likely they are to move into your vessel walls. And the smaller and denser the HDLs are, the less efficient they are at removing the cholesterol from those vessel walls. These changes are also associated with high blood fat levels measured in the form of triglycerides. The fact that these fats are in your bloodstream longer also favours their accumulation in the vessel walls.

So if you have gained predominantly belly fat as an adult and there is diabetes in your family (even if it occurred in a parent or grandparent late in life), you probably are insulin resistant and have prediabetes.

The diagnosis of prediabetes is made if you meet three of the five following criteria:

- **Central obesity:** A waist circumference of greater than 102 cm (40 in) for men and 89 cm (35 in) for women

- **Elevated triglycerides:** Greater than or equal to 1.7 mmol/L

- **Low total HDL:** Less than or equal to 1.0 mmol/L for men and less than or equal to 1.3 mmol/L for women

- **Elevated blood pressure:** Systolic blood pressure of greater than or equal to 130 mm Hg and diastolic blood pressure of greater than or equal to 85 mm Hg

- **Elevated fasting glucose:** Greater than or equal to 5.6 mmol/L

Type 2 diabetes is diagnosed when your pancreas fails to produce enough insulin to overcome the insulin resistance of the bloated fat cells and your fasting blood sugar increases to greater than or equal to 7 mmol/L. With weight loss and exercise, belly fat cells can shrink, allowing for the more efficient use of insulin. In this way, both pre-diabetes and diabetes can often be reversed. However, the stress on the pancreas to produce that extra insulin can reach a point where the pancreas literally burns out. At this point, it cannot produce enough insulin, even after weight loss. Therefore, it is critically important to begin lifestyle changes as early as possible.

Why didn't we know all this earlier? Actually, we've known about diabetes since antiquity because the high levels of sugar in type 1 diabetics' blood spilled over into their urine, which smelled sweet. People with diabetes would literally waste away because not enough sugar and fat entered their tissues to supply the needed calories. (In type 2 diabetes, this rarely happens, because sufficient insulin is produced to move sufficient calories to the cells.) But even though we've been able to measure blood sugar levels for many decades now, the changes in blood fats that also occur were not recognized until recently.

One reason for this is that we used to rely solely on a fasting total cholesterol test to determine blood fat (lipid) levels. The trouble was, the fasting test did not tell the whole story. It would give an accurate reading of total cholesterol, but not of triglycerides, which would be back to or near normal after an overnight fast. That's because in the prediabetic stage, insulin would eventually do its job and clear the blood of sugar and fat, although there could be a delay of several hours. Until recently, we didn't appreciate the significance of nonfasting lipids. When occasionally we did a nonfasting test and saw the elevated triglycerides after eating, we discounted the results.

Moreover, before advanced blood testing, the standard cholesterol tests didn't measure the different sizes of cholesterol. And so, as the LDL and HDL particles shrank and became more dangerous, the total cholesterol level fell, which we thought was a good thing!

All of this threw us off. In fact, the prediabetes syndrome, initially named Syndrome X, was first reported by Dr Gerald Reaven in the late 1980s. It's only in the last decade that we have connected the dots and finally understood why so many people in this country and around the world are becoming prediabetic and diabetic.

Ironically, the disease that is killing us today results from three survival mechanisms that were crucial to early man's existence. These survival mechanisms worked well in the natural environments in which we lived for more than a million years, but they are counter-productive in the modern world of fast food. They are: (1) a tendency to store fat; (2) a desire for sugar, fat and salt; and (3) the ability to adapt to starvation by slowing metabolism. Let's look at these survival mechanisms in the environments of then and now.

A Tendency to Store Fat

The first and perhaps most important survival mechanism is our ability to store fat. From our earliest days on earth, our human ancestors were hunter-gatherers whose existence revolved around hunting and foraging for food. (The cultivation of crops began only some 10,000 years ago.) Because early humans were forced to eat what was available in their immediate surroundings, they regularly experienced cycles of feast and famine. They were also at the mercy of the weather: in warm weather, food was usually plentiful, but in cold weather, it was usually scarce. When there was lots of food to go around, early man consumed more of it and stored excess calories as belly fat. As the belly fat cells enlarged, it resulted in insulin resistance and exaggerated swings in blood sugar. This caused man to become hungrier and store even more belly fat. The belly fat acted like a reserve tank of petrol, which was called upon in the winter or in times of famine. This is in fact how our DNA was designed long ago, and it has not changed significantly in modern times.

The problem – at least in the West – is that we rarely experience famine. It's feast time year-round, so we continue to store fat in our belly and elsewhere. This swells our belly fat cells even more, causing more insulin resistance, greater swings in blood sugar, more hunger, and more fat storage. It becomes a vicious cycle. Today, about 1 in 4 people in the UK between the ages of 40 and 74 are prediabetic. That means they are walking around having big swings in blood sugar and are hungry a lot of the time. No wonder everything is 'supersized'.

Some of you may have seen the 2004 movie *Super Size Me,* in which filmmaker Morgan Spurlock documents the changes that occurred in his health while he was living exclusively on fast food for an entire month. The documentary is an excellent illustration of our fat-storing survival mechanism. At the beginning of the movie, Spurlock was a trim, energetic young man in excellent health. After 6 days of consuming meals consisting of huge burgers and giant orders of fries washed down with bucket-size containers of cola, Spurlock had gained a whopping 4.5 kg (10 lb). After 3 weeks on this diet, he began to complain about food cravings. This signalled the point at which his belly fat cells had reached the size where they were resistant to the action of insulin. The result: exaggerated swings in his blood sugar along with other hormonal changes. By the end of 4 weeks, Spurlock looked and felt like a total wreck. He had developed the telltale belly fat typical of prediabetes, his cholesterol had soared 1.3 mmol/L, and his energy level and libido had crashed.

Our genetic predisposition to store fat has been called the *thrifty gene theory.* What I find fascinating about the thrifty gene today is that it appears to most strongly manifest itself in societies that have experienced starvation in recent times. One example, well known to researchers, is the story of the Pima Indians. They survived in the desert of the southwestern United States on a subsistence diet until fairly recently. Starvation was always a threat. For them, the ability to efficiently store fat was crucial for survival. Their thrifty gene served them well until they graduated from their subsistence diet to a Western diet, along with a more sedentary lifestyle, a few decades ago. They now experience almost universal obesity, and more than 50 per cent of the Pima population develops diabetes by the age of 40. Even worse, their children are obese and developing type 2 diabetes at a record pace. The Pima Indians are also racked by premature heart attacks and strokes as a result of their thrifty gene being combined with a poor diet.

Other groups that have experienced subsistence living in recent times also appear to be more prone to obesity, diabetes and heart disease when their diets are Westernized. The Chinese and Asians are examples. As we export our fast-food lifestyle to societies around the world, we are seeing a global increase in these serious ailments.

Following Our Taste Buds

The second survival mechanism that worked well for the health of the hunter-gatherers but isn't helping the health of modern man is our desire for sweet, fatty and salty foods.

The desire for sweetness led hunter-gatherers to seek out a healthy variety of nutrient- and fibre-rich fruits and vegetables. But because they also ate significantly more fibre than we do today (it was present in the fruits and vegetables), they didn't suffer from insulin resistance. Fibre is one of nature's ways of preventing insulin resistance. It slows down the digestion of carbohydrates, preventing the rapid spike in blood sugar levels that can cause reactive hypoglycaemia, food cravings, and ultimately the insulin resistance that leads to diabetes.

It was the hunter-gatherers' desire for fat that led them to regularly risk their lives in search of big game, which contained tasty, mouth-watering fat. Back then, the fat in big-game meat did not look like the marbled steaks we get in supermarkets and restaurants today. It was rich in anti-inflammatory, heart-healthy omega-3s (from the indigenous grasses the animals thrived on), and it also had much less saturated fat than that from today's grain-fed, sedentary cattle.

Finally, the hunter-gatherers' innate desire for salt also helped them survive. Today we know that sodium is necessary in order to maintain the body's fluid volume; without adequate sodium intake, we would become dehydrated and die. But salt is an example of something that in larger amounts can be too much of a good thing: excess sodium intake in the form of salt is an important risk factor for high blood pressure. Societies with low levels of salt intake (comparable to that of the hunter-gatherers) do not have the age-related increase in blood pressure and decrease in kidney function seen in the Western world.

Ironically, the desire for sweet, fatty and salty foods that led our ancestors to a highly nutritious diet is what leads contemporary men, women and children straight to nutrient-poor fast food. This is an important reason why many Westerners, while seemingly overfed, are actually undernourished.

We're No Longer Made for Extremes

The third survival mechanism that wreaks havoc with today's dieters is the decrease in our metabolism that occurs when we are on a severely restricted low-calorie diet; it's comparable to the slowdown people experience when they are starving. I often tell my patients and friends that if they've had problems with yo-yo dieting (meaning that they lose weight quickly, gain it back again, and then have to lose it all over again, only to gain back even more weight later), it's because our metabolism was not made for rapid weight loss.

For early man, who would regularly go through a period of famine and consequent weight loss, a decrease in metabolism meant fewer calories were necessary for survival. Man survived the famine by getting by on less food. This is, in fact, the way we humans are designed. When we drastically reduce our caloric intake, we eventually burn

INFLAMMATION: THE BANE OF CIVILIZATION

Inflammation is another important survival mechanism that was as critical for our hunter-gatherer ancestors as it is today. Life was dangerous for early man, and injury was a common occurrence. If you were bitten by a wild animal in the forest or you cut yourself in the process of capturing and skinning your dinner, you would die unless two things happened. First, your blood had to clot quickly so you didn't bleed to death. Second, your immune system had to be activated to make sure that your wound did not become infected.

What I've just described is the body's inflammatory response to injury. On the one hand, it's a good thing, because it helps the body respond quickly to assaults. On the other hand, it's a bad thing when it's kept on chronically, because the inflammatory response can begin to hurt healthy cells and tissues such as the endothelial lining of the coronary arteries. This is how chronic inflammation contributes to heart attacks.

The problem is that, due to our current poor diet and sedentary lifestyle, many of us are continually in a hyperinflammatory state. The most commonly used measure of this state is a protein called *C-reactive protein*, or CRP, which we measure with a simple blood test (see page 206).

So why am I including a discussion of inflammation in a chapter on our waistlines? It turns out that inflammation, as reflected by elevated CRP, is associated with belly fat. This is because the inflammatory response requires quite a bit of energy. If you do not have a reserve of at least some belly fat, you cannot afford this energy expenditure. That's why starving people, who lack fat stores, cannot mount an inflammatory response. Such malnourished individuals are well known to be particularly susceptible to infection. Normal fat stores mean a normal inflammatory response.

The problem today is that we are carrying around an unprecedented reserve of belly fat – much more than was ever needed by our ancestors for survival. This excess fat produces chronic inflammation, which contributes to diabetes and heart disease, and is also thought to be a factor in cancer, Alzheimer's disease, macular degeneration, arthritis and many other diseases of modern civilization. Following the healthy eating principles I outline in Step 1 of the South Beach Heart Programme can go a long way towards reducing belly fat and countering harmful inflammation.

protein from muscle and bone to maintain our blood sugar. Muscle requires more calories to be maintained than fat does. When we have less muscle, we burn fewer calories, even while we are at rest. The amount of calories we need at rest is called our *basal metabolic rate*.

How does this slowdown in metabolism affect modern dieters who desire quick weight loss? When today's crash dieters lose weight too fast, especially without exercising (which builds muscle and bone mass in addition to its cardiovascular and calorie-burning benefits), they lose muscle and activate the survival mechanism that decreases their metabolic rate. Weight loss slows and then stops, and when the dieters return to their usual diet, they end up gaining the weight they lost and then some. Thus, losing weight too rapidly and not exercising becomes counterproductive and leads to the classic yo-yo syndrome.

I hope that by understanding our inherent survival mechanisms, you can better understand what we are up against in our modern, unnatural, fast-food environment. The first step in reversing our often-toxic lifestyle is gaining a good understanding of how we got here. While modern times and technology have improved our lives for the most part, they have also had important adverse affects on our health. The good news is that we do have a much better understanding than ever before of the causes of obesity, diabetes, heart disease and other chronic diseases of the Western world. This gives us the opportunity to develop effective strategies to improve our health and longevity.

6

EVERY PICTURE TELLS A STORY

On the outside, John appeared to be the picture of health to his doctors and friends. The 46-year-old lawyer and triathlete ran several miles every morning, swam lengths at night, and kept flexible with Pilates. John, who had heart disease on both sides of his family, took fitness very seriously and it showed. His lean, muscular body was the envy of his friends and colleagues, many of whom were beginning to show the telltale paunch of middle age. John's numbers were 'normal' – his total cholesterol was under 5.2 mmol/L and his HDL cholesterol and LDL cholesterol were within the normal range. His blood pressure was an enviable 115/75. But on the inside, things were beginning to go terribly wrong.

One morning, after running only a few blocks, John was so out of breath he had to sit down. The next morning, when he tried to run again, he broke out in a sweat and felt a tightness in his chest. My friend Mark, who happened to be John's law partner, suggested that he call me. I agreed to see John immediately, but when he arrived at the hospital, his story and his electrocardiogram showed that he had already experienced a heart attack. I sent him directly to the cath lab for an angiogram, hoping that the blockage causing his symptoms could be opened with angioplasty and at least some heart muscle could be saved. Unfortunately, a simple angioplasty was not technically feasible. John had multiple blockages in his coronary arteries and went directly to bypass surgery.

Soon after John's surgery, Mark called me in a panic. The consensus in the law firm was that 'If John could go down, any one of us could go down. You've got to help him…and us.' We ended up doing advanced blood testing and heart scans on about 30 members of the law firm and found that two lawyers, though they didn't know it, were at very high risk for a heart attack. Others had varying degrees of risk, but these two were heart attacks waiting to happen. I am now treating Mark and his high-risk partners.

A few months after John's surgery, I performed a CT heart scan on him as a baseline so I could monitor his future progress (for more on this test, see pages 208–10). We already knew from his angiogram that he had extensive plaque. From the scan, I could see that his arteries, as expected, had extensive calcified plaque consistent with the atherosclerosis that had already been diagnosed.

Taking the Guesswork Out of Medicine

My frustration with John's case (and many similar cases I see, hear about, or read about) was that his heart attack and his surgery could have been prevented. Had John had a heart scan 1, 2, 5 or even 10 years earlier, we could have seen his silent atherosclerosis and realized his heightened risk for a future heart attack right then, even though he apparently was in outstanding health. The earlier the disease could have been detected, the greater the chance of success. Even a simple aspirin daily could have decreased his heart attack risk by 25 per cent. The good news is that John survived the bypass and, although a large amount of heart muscle was involved, much of it has recovered.

Six years later, John has an excellent quality of life and is still exercising regularly and vigorously. What's more, a recent heart scan showed that his atherosclerotic process is stable and his bypass grafts are free of plaque.

Had I seen John years ago without the benefit of a heart scan, I, too, would have thought that he was in spectacular shape. But, given his family history, I would have had concerns. Should I simply have told him that he was looking great and that he should keep up the good work? Given the possibility that he had a hidden problem due to unknown risk factors running in his family, should I have reached for my prescription pad and put him on strong drugs for the rest of his life, even though he may not have needed them? His lipid profile numbers did not meet the national guidelines for beginning medications – then or now. Without knowing what his arteries actually looked like, I would have had to make a decision based on incomplete information – and I could well have made the wrong one.

Window of Opportunity

The point I want to make here is that if a man in his mid-forties like John is heading for a heart attack – whether it's in 1, 5 or 15 years – he will already have built up coronary atherosclerotic plaque. How do we know this? Numerous autopsy studies show that atherosclerosis begins early, as early as a person's late teens or early twenties. The problem for those of us interested in early detection of heart disease is that both men *and women* may have been building up plaque for years *without symptoms*.

The critical lesson to be learned is that there is a big window of opportunity – a long period of time – to discover and treat atherosclerotic plaque before it causes chest pain or a heart attack. If we wait until a patient experiences symptoms to begin treatment, we will have waited until severe, and potentially lethal, disease has developed.

The Relationship between Plaque and Risk Factors

As noted in Chapter 2, patients we see in coronary care units often don't have many of the conventional risk factors that put them at high risk for a heart attack. Doing advanced blood testing helps us figure out who these high-risk people are, but both known and yet-to-be-discovered risk factors mix differently in each patient. Depending on how they mix, each individual will have his or her own *cholesterol threshold* where cholesterol is effectively entering the vessel walls and building up plaque. Fortunately, it has been clearly shown that if you have plaque, lowering your cholesterol further will slow or stop its progression – no matter how low or high your initial cholesterol levels were. This is why it is so critical for us to identify those people who are developing plaque at an early enough stage to effectively intervene.

Imaging Plaque

Two types of noninvasive heart scans are now widely used. The first, the coronary calcium scan, is performed in minutes without a dye injection. The second, called a *noninvasive angiogram*, requires an intravenous dye injection. It images coronary calcium as well as soft plaque. Both methods give you your Calcium Score (also known as the Agatston Score), which, as I noted earlier, tells you how much hard, calcified plaque you have accumulated in your arteries. The Calcium Score is the best single predictor of who is destined for a heart attack in the future. The higher your Calcium Score, the higher your risk.

In addition to your total Calcium Score, the scan report will also tell you how much plaque you have compared to others of your own age and sex. This extra information gives you an idea not only of how much plaque you have, but also how fast it is accumulating. For example, if you are 50 years old and have a Calcium Score of 100, your atherosclerosis is progressing much more rapidly than a 70-year-old with a Calcium Score of 100 (in whom it has taken 20 more years to develop the same amount of plaque). This difference will be reflected in what is called your *Percentile Score*. A 50-year-old male with a Calcium Score of 100 is in the 75th percentile of risk. In other words, he has more plaque than 75 per cent of men his age. The 70-year-old has a Percentile Score of 40 per cent, indicating that he has less plaque than most men his age. His atherosclerosis is progressing much more slowly than the 50-year-old's, even though he has accumulated the same total amount of plaque. The amount of calcified plaque you have at any given time reflects what has developed over your entire lifetime.

If you improve your risk factors for heart disease with lifestyle changes and medications, you can slow your Calcium Score progression to about a 10 per cent increase per year. Yes, I said *slow*, not *stop*. Many of my patients who are diligently following my aggressive prevention programme get very worried when their Calcium Score increases, even if it's at a much slower rate than 10 per cent a year. I tell them not to worry. *The slight increase in a Calcium Score does not reflect new plaque formation, but rather an increase in the density of the scar tissue that forms when a ruptured plaque heals.*

Over the many years I have practised cardiology, I have observed ever-accelerating technological advancement. In my own area of non-invasive cardiac imaging, for example, the progress in cardiac ultrasound, cardiac magnetic resonance imaging (MRI), and cardiac CT scans has been particularly exciting. The most recent major advance in heart imaging is the 64-slice CT scanner, which is ideal for performing the noninvasive angiogram. In contrast to the invasive angiogram (catheterization), the 64-slice scan is done from completely outside the body, and nothing could be simpler. In fact, from a patient's perspective, a heart scan is easy. It's so easy, in fact, that you don't have to get out of your clothes or skip breakfast before having the procedure. You can get a heart scan during your lunch break and be back to work on time. The fact that it is safe, fast and noninvasive makes it an ideal screening tool. For more specifics on how the scan is actually done, see pages 208–10 in Step 3 of the programme.

What Has Your Doctor Done for You Lately?

I do not want to get too technical, so let's just say that with the 64-slice scan, we can for the first time reliably image *soft* plaque non-invasively. Why is this so important? By imaging the amount of soft plaque you have and comparing a baseline heart scan to subsequent

(*continued on page 88*)

A BIT OF HISTORY

In May 1988, while I was director of the noninvasive cardiac lab at Mount Sinai Medical Center in Miami Beach, Florida, David King, the director of clinical science with what was then the Imatron Corporation, came to my office to try to convince me of the value of the new high-speed electron-beam tomography (EBT) scanner. The new EBT scanner, which Mount Sinai had installed a year before, provided some excellent views of the beating heart, but there wasn't enough use for the machine to justify its cost. In fact, Mount Sinai was ready to return the scanner because we could get similar information using less expensive technology, such as ultrasound.

As David showed me the different features of the EBT scanner, he pointed out something that caught my interest: he told me that the EBT scanner could be many times more sensitive than fluoroscopy (a form of x-ray) at detecting calcium in vessels. Immediately, a lightbulb turned on in my brain. I knew from autopsy studies that coronary calcium was intimately associated with coronary atherosclerosis. It was the calcium component of plaque in the heart's vessels that caused the 'hardening' of the arteries.

I was also aware of studies that showed a direct relationship between the amount of calcium and the total amount of atherosclerosis in the coronary arteries. At this point, the first statin drugs had become available. We could, for the first time, decrease cholesterol levels dramatically. The question I thought needed answering was 'Who would be the best candidates for these wonder drugs?' I had already learned that using only high cholesterol as a criterion for treatment excluded too many patients destined for heart attacks. I thought that noninvasively imaging and quantifying plaque using calcium as a marker could tell us who needed to be treated with the statins.

I immediately called radiologist Warren Janowitz for help. In short order, we came up with a protocol to image coronary calcium. David King volunteered to be the first patient, and the images of his coronary arteries amazed us. The only problem was that David didn't have any calcium – and neither did Warren or I. Several other doctors volunteered, and we soon saw plenty of coronary calcium. The images were exquisite.

Now that we knew that we could see calcium so well, the next step was to find a way to attach a number to reflect the total amount. Dr Janowitz and I sat down to come up with a *Calcium Score*. This was rather crude, but it has stood the test of time. A few years later, at a meeting in Hilton Head, South Carolina, I was surprised to hear someone refer to the *Agatston Score*, because I was the first author on the first paper describing the heart scan and coronary calcium. I've always felt that the name *Agatston-Janowitz Score* or *Agatston-Janowitz-King Score* would have been more accurate. (Sadly, David King passed away from cancer in 2004.)

In our first study using our Calcium Score, which was published in 1990 in the *Journal of the American College of Cardiology,* Dr Janowitz and I, along with other colleagues, demonstrated that patients who had sustained heart attacks or had coronary artery blockages had much higher Calcium Scores than those without clinical disease. Several other studies followed. These included research from the Mayo Clinic that showed that in autopsied coronary arteries, the amount of calcium detected on heart scans closely correlated with the total amount of plaque in the arteries. We were very excited by these findings.

Knowing that heart attacks were caused by atherosclerosis, we hypothesized that if we could quantify the amount of atherosclerosis using the Calcium Score, it might be a good predictor of heart attacks. But not everyone jumped on board. I was amazed by the resistance shown by many in the medical and research community to this seemingly simple hypothesis. I felt that much of the scepticism was due to an overall orientation towards intervention rather than prevention. Luckily that tide is changing, and it must continue to change if we are ever to make a dent in heart disease.

Today, there have been dramatic advances in the heart scan, notably the 64-slice CT scanner described in this chapter and on pages 208–9. This scanner combines scanning speed and resolution to produce images of the coronary arteries that are better than ever before. In fact, it's the best way to image coronary soft plaque noninvasively.

With continued technological progress, even better scanners are in the pipeline. I have always felt that whatever we can't see well this year, we will be able to see better next year with the next generation of software and hardware. The future of preventing heart disease with the help of this new technology looks very bright.

scans, we can tell a lot about how your risk factors are interacting with your arteries. What I often tell my patients is that seeing the presence or absence of soft plaque is evidence of what I have done for you lately. It also tells you what you have done for yourself lately. For example, if your risk has increased abruptly, possibly because you stopped exercising and gained weight over the course of a year or so, you might be developing soft plaque where you had very little previously, and we will see it on the scan.

With this new information readily available, practising cardiology has become more rewarding than ever before. I can easily see for myself how you are doing and also show you the results of our combined preventive efforts.

Heart Scans Save Lives

Currently, the guidelines on heart scans from US organizations suggest that the scans have value for people at moderate risk for whom there is a question of whether or not to treat with cholesterol-lowering medications. The US Society of Atherosclerosis Imaging and Prevention recommends a heart scan for men over the age of 45 and women over the age of 55 who have risk factors for cardiovascular disease, including any of the risks I described in Chapter 3. The American Heart Association recognizes the heart scan as a potentially useful tool for people who are at moderate risk, but stops short of recommending it. There are no formal guidelines in the UK, however, and heart scans are not routinely available on the NHS.

In July 2006, the US Screening for Heart Attack Prevention and Education (SHAPE) task-force report, from a prominent group of heart specialists affiliated with the Association for Eradication of Heart Attack (AEHA), took a bold step forwards in the fight against heart disease. The report, published in the *American Journal of Cardiology*, recommended CT scans for measuring coronary artery calcium and/or carotid ultrasound for *all* at-risk asymptomatic men between the ages of 45 and 75 and *all* at-risk asymptomatic women aged 55 to 75.

At the present time, most private health insurance companies view a heart scan as a tool for heart disease screening, not treatment, so they usually do not cover the test. This could change as more medical authorities recognize the lifesaving and money-saving potential of heart scanning technology. For now, you will most likely have to pay for your heart scan out of your own pocket. But the good news is that the cost is now within the reach of most people. Getting a heart scan can cost less than buying a flat-screen TV or purchasing new tyres for your car.

I like to think of the heart scan as the 'mammogram of the heart' and believe that if it is widely used as a screening tool, like the mammogram, it will save many lives. My preference would be to perform at least a baseline heart scan on all men over 40 who have any risk factors for heart disease and on all women over 50 who are postmenopausal and have any risk factors. This simple, noninvasive procedure would identify a large number of people with otherwise unrecognized atherosclerosis and make it possible to begin treatment years before a problem arises. For patients with little or no plaque buildup (reflected in a low Calcium Score), the test should be repeated every 5 years. For patients with signs of plaque buildup, the test should be repeated every 2 to 5 years depending on other risk factors.

A Heart Crisis That Shouldn't Have Happened

There is no better example of the inadequacy of standard heart screening procedures than the heart history of former US president Bill Clinton. President Clinton was known for his love of rich foods, especially fatty foods like hamburgers, doughnuts, fried pie and fried chicken. To his credit, he was also an avid jogger and ran 5 miles several times a week. For many years, it appeared that the exercise was helping to compensate for his appetite. He seemed reasonably fit and healthy.

In January 2001, the 54-year-old Clinton was given his sixth and final presidential physical exam. As in his previous physicals, he was examined for several hours by a panel of medical experts at Bethesda Naval Hospital. During the press briefing that followed, the

MAKING SENSE OF YOUR CALCIUM SCORE

When you have a heart scan, you are given an overall number called the Calcium Score, or Agatston Score, which represents the total amount of plaque in your coronary arteries. The number can range from 0 to 1000 or more. The higher your number, the more plaque you have in your arteries and the greater your risk. If your score is more than 400, for example, you have an increased likelihood of developing symptomatic heart disease – angina, heart attack or even sudden death – in the next 2 to 5 years. *If your score is more than 1000, you have a 25 per cent chance of having a heart attack within a year without intervention.*

Calcium Score for a 55-Year-Old Man or Woman	Relative Amount of Plaque
0–10	Minimal
11–100	Moderate
101–400	Increased
401+	Extensive

Keep in mind that there's no absolute way to predict who is going to have a heart attack, but your Calcium Score is an excellent way of predicting the likelihood of it happening to you. Of course, when you are trying to predict the future, you must consider other variables beyond your Calcium Score. For example, if you smoke, a low Calcium Score will not protect you. Smokers tend to have very sticky blood. This can result in a much larger blood clot developing after a plaque rupture than would develop in a nonsmoker. On the other hand, someone with a moderately high Calcium Score can forestall a heart attack indefinitely – or even prevent one entirely – simply by controlling risk factors. And even if your Calcium Score indicates a high likelihood for a heart attack in the near future, if you begin an aggressive prevention pro-gramme immediately, your level of risk can sharply decline within months.

president's personal doctor said that he had passed and had a 'fairly normal exam'. There was only one heart health problem worth mentioning. The president's LDL cholesterol had gone up from 3.5 to 4.6 mmol/L, which was high according to national standards. He was prescribed simvastatin (Zocor), a well-known cholesterol-lowering medication, and advised to be more vigilant about his diet and exercise.

Today we know that when President Clinton was given that exam, he had extensive plaque throughout his coronary arteries and was at high risk for a heart attack. The diagnostic tool that would have revealed the seriousness of his condition was a heart scan, and it would have taken 10 minutes or less. For want of a scan, President Clinton, arguably then the most influential person in the world, left Bethesda Naval Hospital a cardiac time bomb.

It took 3 years for the fuse to ignite. When Clinton resumed civilian life, he continued to jog, but found he could no longer run 5 miles. He blamed it on the fact that he had been too busy to exercise during much of his second term. He thought that he just needed to get back in shape.

In an effort to lose weight, he went on the South Beach Diet, and he actually did get back down to his high school weight. This was an important step in the right direction, but not enough to undo the past damage. He also continued to take Zocor for many months, but, like many people, he unfortunately stopped taking it as soon as his cholesterol dropped to an acceptable level due to the combination of weight loss and medication. If he had known the true condition of his arteries, he would have stayed on the statin and probably added other medications as well.

On August 31, 2004, President Clinton was returning home from a trip to New Orleans. As he got off the plane, he felt a severe tightness in his chest. It was something he had experienced several times before, but only during exercise. This time, it was more alarming. He called his doctor, who told him to go to the hospital for tests. He was given an angiogram, which revealed that he had severe blockage in multiple coronary arteries. Unfortunately, it took a near heart attack to alert the president and his doctors to the fact that he had advanced cardiovascular disease. As soon as it could be arranged, he underwent quadruple bypass surgery at Manhattan's New York-Presbyterian Hospital/ Columbia University Medical Center.

The lesson to be learned from President Clinton's experience is that conventional heart screening tests – even when administered by the best doctors in the land – do a poor job of predicting what is going on in your coronary arteries. A 2003 study published in the *Journal of the American College of Cardiology* drives this point home. Researchers examined the medical records of 222 heart attack victims. They concluded that if the victims had been given the standard screening tests for heart disease the day before the attack occurred, only 25 per cent of them would have been classified as being high-risk patients who needed therapy. The remaining 75 per cent would have been given a clean bill of health and sent home with no treatment whatsoever.

In the period since President Clinton's ordeal, heart scanning has become more common and is proving to be unsurpassed in detecting 'hidden' cases of coronary artery disease. With each passing year, the procedure has gradually become less expensive and more widely available.

Seeing Is Complying

In addition to using heart scans to help diagnose cardiovascular disease, doctors can use them to monitor how well their patients are responding to medications. Instead of asking the indirect question 'Is my patient's cholesterol low enough?' they can ask the more useful question 'Does my patient have more or less plaque than he or she did 2 years ago?' This more precise information can help doctors fine-tune a patient's therapy.

A heart scan can also be a powerful motivator for patients. Currently, only about half of patients continue to take statins after just 1 year. However, when patients have a heart scan and see the amount of plaque in their arteries with their own eyes, they are much more likely to take statins as prescribed. A recent survey determined that 90 per cent of patients who saw an image of their diseased arteries and who had a Calcium Score over 400 kept taking their cholesterol-lowering medications.

Paul's Story

'Those were my arteries, and they were not looking good.'

My brother had a heart attack 2 years ago. As soon as he recovered, he was after me to go to the doctor and get my cholesterol checked. I figured that I was only 41, 10 years younger than he was, so I had time to think about it. Then my wife got after me. She kept saying that my dad had died of a heart attack at 63, and my brother had a heart attack at 50, and that she didn't want me to be next. At the time, I wasn't doing much about my diet. In fact, I was eating horribly. I just didn't see myself having a heart attack. I wasn't overweight. I played basketball.

Then my wife read something in the paper about Dr Agatston doing advanced testing and begged me to go and see him. I went, and the doctor gave me a new blood test that showed me I had too much LDL cholesterol and that it was the wrong size. He also gave me a heart scan. He told me the results of the scan. My Calcium Score was really high – 720. But what scared me was seeing the actual pictures of my arteries. Two of them were filled with visible white plaque. Those were my arteries, and they were not looking good. I had to accept the fact that I was in the same boat as my brother and father.

Because of the scan, I vowed that my life would be different. I'm now taking two different medications, and I've dramatically changed what I eat. I'm happy to report that my numbers are good and that I'm feeling better than I've ever felt before. ■

7

SHOULD YOU BE TAKING
HEART MEDICATIONS?

When I tell high-risk patients that I think they should take a statin
drug and explain why it will help to improve their cholesterol levels,
they usually agree. But it is not unusual to get some resistance from
patients who aren't well informed about the potential benefits or side
effects of these drugs.

The following are some typical patient reactions:

'No! I don't want to take any medications. I want to lower my
cholesterol naturally, without drugs and their side effects. Won't drugs
fry my liver?'

'Sign me up! I'd rather take a pill than worry about my diet or
bother with exercise!'

In both cases, these patients are just cheating themselves.

Patients who reject medications because they think they're not
'natural' are missing out on some of the best tools in aggressive prevention. Statin drugs alone can slash the risk of having a heart attack
by more than 30 per cent – and by much more than that when taken
in combination with other drugs such as niacin, aspirin and/or certain
blood pressure medications.

I am quick to remind patients who make remarks about drugs not
being 'natural' that there is nothing 'natural' about having a sick
artery that is burdened with plaque. I also tell them that statin drugs
can actually help to restore the artery to its youthful, flexible state –
the way that nature intended it to be. And I remind them that a truly

'natural' cholesterol level is 3 mmol/L or less. At least that is the level found in populations with unprocessed, non-Western diets.

Patients who think that popping a pill renders diet and exercise unnecessary are also making a deadly mistake. Drugs are meant to work together with these lifestyle changes; they are not meant to replace them. *Even if a combination of drugs can reduce your risk of having a heart attack by 50 per cent, half of all people taking these drugs who were destined for a heart attack will still have one.* That's why making lifestyle changes is so essential to further reduce risk.

Although I am a passionate believer in the power of diet and exercise, given what we know today about the effectiveness of statins and other drugs, it makes no sense at all for at-risk patients not to take them. I made this point recently when I was lecturing at a major medical centre about the benefits of good fats, good carbs and lean protein to a group of doctors. At the end of my talk, after having built a strong case for the role of diet in heart disease prevention, one doctor asked if I would be willing to conduct a study that tested the principles of the South Beach Diet as a sole therapy for patients with coronary artery disease. I was adamant that I would not. Using diet alone to treat heart disease would be ignoring 30 years of lifesaving medical advances.

So does that mean that statins should be universally prescribed in a manner akin to adding fluoride to drinking water to reduce tooth decay? That would be going too far. But statins have generally been underprescribed. Despite numerous excellent studies documenting their effectiveness, millions of people who should be taking these cholesterol-lowering

A WORD OF CAUTION

Tell your doctor about all the medications and dietary supplements you take regularly, whether they're prescription or over-the-counter. When taken in combination with other drugs, many otherwise safe medications can interact, causing potentially dangerous side effects. Never stop taking a heart medication without consulting your doctor.

drugs are not. This means that millions of people have an unnecessarily high risk of suffering a heart attack, stroke or sudden death.

A Tale of Two Brothers

I'm not suggesting that everyone needs to take a statin to prevent heart disease. In some cases, if a high-risk patient is still young, I allow 3 months to a year to see if diet, exercise and other lifestyle modifications can make enough difference to avoid medications. Today, thanks to heart scans and advanced blood testing, we can more precisely identify those people who *will* benefit from taking a statin.

Let me tell you about two brothers, Chuck, 34 years old, and Steven, 36 years old, who came to me because their father had suffered a heart attack at the young age of 49. Both brothers wanted to do everything they could to avoid their father's fate.

I did heart scans and advanced blood testing on both brothers. Chuck's scan showed that his arteries already had plaque; with a Calcium Score in the 20s at the young age of 34, it meant his risk of having a future heart attack was high for his age. Furthermore, his advanced blood tests showed that he had high amounts of small, dense LDL, the really bad cholesterol, and low amounts of HDL, the good cholesterol. In comparison, his brother Steven's arteries were picture-perfect – and so were his blood tests. Unlike Chuck, Steven had probably inherited his mother's healthier genes.

Chuck left my office with a prescription for atorvastatin (Lipitor), a statin drug, to lower his bad LDL cholesterol, as well as one for niacin, which helps reduce the production of small LDL cholesterol and raise HDL. Chuck was also given nutrition counselling and exercise advice. Lucky Steven didn't need to do anything other than follow a heart-healthy diet and exercise regime.

Chuck's case required what in my medical practice we call a 'full-court press'. His risk was so high, and there was such a clear genetic component to his problem, that he deserved every antiplaque weapon we had in our arsenal. And, of course, he still needed to be conscientious with regard to diet and exercise.

More Cases in Point

I have other patients with very bad family histories of premature heart disease who have come to me *after* a cardiac event. Because of their histories, these patients had made every effort to lead healthy lives. And yet they still developed either angina or heart attacks. As it happened, these events occurred later than they had in other family members, so their exemplary lifestyles did indeed slow their progression of atherosclerosis – but didn't stop it.

Years ago, in the pre-statin 1980s, I heard a case presentation made by Dr Bill Roberts, a famous cardiac pathologist. He showed the autopsy of a congressman who had tragically died while jogging at the age of 55. There was extensive plaque buildup in all of the politician's major coronary arteries. Dr Roberts remarked that the congressman was a regular long-distance runner and that he had outlived his siblings by a full 10 years due to his vigorous regular exercise routine and his strict diet. But despite his best efforts to fight his genetics with lifestyle alone, it wasn't good enough. If he had received the benefit of early diagnosis and the best of our current medications to complement his exemplary lifestyle, I am confident he could have survived to a ripe old age.

But Will Statins Really Help?

Initially, there was some doubt about whether statins would be helpful to anyone other than a small number of patients who were genetically predisposed to very high total cholesterol levels.

Studies conducted in the early 1990s, however, produced some very exciting findings. For example, the landmark 5-year Scandinavian Simvastatin Survival Study (4S) of 4444 Scandinavian heart patients who were taking simvastatin (Zocor) showed that they had a 34 per cent reduction in their risk of dying from heart-related causes and a 37 per cent reduction in their chances of undergoing angioplasty or bypass surgery. This was a momentous study because it demonstrated for the first time that a cholesterol-lowering drug had reduced the need for surgery and saved a significant number of lives. Statins were no longer promising – they were proven.

Since then, statins have been studied in dozens of other large and small clinical trials involving tens of thousands of people. One of the newest findings is that when high-dose statins are used to drop LDL cholesterol to very low levels – 1.8 mmol/L or less – there appears to be an even greater reduction in the number of heart attacks, strokes and sudden deaths.

And there's more good news about statins. Besides lowering cholesterol, these drugs attack cardiovascular disease on other fronts as well, by calming inflammation, fighting cell-damaging free radicals, and, most importantly, by making vulnerable soft plaque regress and less likely to rupture. As you know from what I've said in earlier chapters, plaque rupture is the event that triggers most heart attacks and strokes. The fact that statins do so much more than merely lower cholesterol explains why these drugs are prescribed immediately following a coronary event. In fact, it is now recommended that heart attack patients begin a statin while they are still in the hospital. All told, statins are more effective in managing atherosclerosis and preventing heart attack, stroke and death than all other classes of medicine.

But Are Statins Safe?

Contrary to what you may have heard, today's statin medications are quite safe. The only serious side effect I have ever seen was an acute breakdown in muscle that can lead to kidney failure and death, which occurred with cerivastatin (Baycol). In 2001, Baycol was taken off the market. While this side effect is reported with other statins, it is exceedingly rare, and if recognized early, it is completely reversible. I personally have never observed this complication with any of the statins I currently prescribe.

In fact, in five major studies involving 30,817 patients who were prescribed statins, only one person had a severe muscle complication, and there were no cases of serious liver disease, another potential side effect. The only problems with statins that I do see fairly commonly are muscle aches and pains and occasionally muscle cramps, particularly in the toes. I have found that switching a patient to a different statin drug or altering the dosage often helps. These harmless aches and pains are *not* a sign of the serious muscle complication just described. However, do tell your doctor if you are having any muscle pain.

Cholesterol – How Low Should It Go?

If you have established heart disease or are at high risk, aggressive cholesterol lowering is beneficial no matter what cholesterol levels you start with. There are a number of studies that demonstrate this.

In fact, one of the five statin studies referred to above, the 1998 Air Force/Texas Atherosclerosis Coronary Prevention Study, was different from prior statin investigations. In this study, the participants started with normal levels of total and LDL ('bad') cholesterol and no obvious signs of cardiovascular disease. Understandably, many people thought that giving statins to people with normal LDL cholesterol was 'overkill'. In truth, it turned out to be lifesaving. Compared to people who were given a sugar pill (placebo), those who took a statin had a 37 per cent lower risk of having a heart attack, unstable angina or sudden cardiac death.

A more recent study, the 5-year Heart Protection Study, reported in 2002, backed up these results. In this study, a statin was given to half of 20,536 subjects with risk factors for heart disease other than a bad LDL cholesterol level. In fact, some of the study volunteers had a relatively good level of LDL (below 3 mmol/L) to begin with. The results showed that cholesterol-lowering statin therapy decreased heart attacks equally in those starting with an LDL level of less than 3 mmol/L and in those who had a higher initial level of LDL.

In yet another study, published in 2005 and known as the 'PROVE-IT trial', more than 4000 patients with an elevated LDL cholesterol level who were hospitalized for either a heart attack or unstable angina were given one of two statin drugs and followed for up to 2 years. In one group, LDL levels were decreased to less than 1.8 mmol/L, as compared with a decrease to about 2.6 mmol/L in the other group. Those who had their LDL lowered to at least 1.8 mmol/L had significantly fewer cardiac events, and there was even further incremental benefit as the LDL was lowered below 1.5 mmol/L.

Despite these studies, some doctors and researchers believe that using medications to lower cholesterol to very low levels may be dangerous. As far as I'm concerned, there is a danger, but it is from the high levels of cholesterol caused by our modern lifestyle, not the low levels we get by using cholesterol-lowering drugs. Newborns and people living in most pre-industrial societies have a 'normal' total cholesterol level of 3.1 mmol/L or less. In the United States, our 'normal' is about 5.2 mmol/L. In the UK our average total cholesterol level is 5.7 mmol/L. From my perspective, one could say that aggressive statin therapy simply reduces cholesterol to 'natural' levels.

Would You Benefit from Taking a Statin?

How do you know if you would benefit from taking a statin or another cholesterol-lowering medication? This is something you will need to discuss with your doctor. In my practice, I lower my patients' cholesterol levels until I believe I have arrested or reversed the underlying disease. The ultimate level, of course, varies from patient to patient. One patient with an LDL cholesterol of 4.1 mmol/L might have little or no plaque and not require a statin. Another with the very same cholesterol level but a more significant amount of plaque might benefit from aggressive statin treatment.

However, you can get some idea of what your doctor might advise by referring to the guidelines for LDL cholesterol on page 65. As you can see, the higher your LDL level, the greater your risk of having a heart attack or stroke. (You are at the highest risk if you have diabetes or known heart disease.)

Polypharmacy:
Prescribing Multiple Medications

Years ago, during my training, I heard a story about using multiple medications to treat a patient with heart disease. It involved Dr Sam Levine, one of the most famous cardiologists of the 1950s and a medical consultant to President Eisenhower's doctors. As the story goes, Dr Levine was making teaching rounds one day with his usual entourage. After an intern finished presenting a patient who was on many medications, Dr Levine turned to leave with the parting words, 'Stop all but one.' The intern chased after him, asking, 'But which one, Doctor?' To which Levine replied, 'Any one.' This scepticism towards the use of multiple drugs was common back then. And for good reason. The small number of medications we had for treating heart disease (and many other diseases as well) tended to be of limited value. Many of the drugs had serious side effects, especially at the maximum doses often given. And when used in combination, the likelihood of experiencing those side effects only multiplied. But they were the only choices at the time.

Today I can choose from literally scores of medications that are both safe and wonderfully effective. Often we use them in combinations so that the patient takes lower, safer and better-tolerated doses of each individual drug. Most people at high risk for heart disease or stroke do take more than one medication. In fact, some people may take five or six or more. Critics are quick to call this over-medication, and there is indeed some cause for concern.

However, when medications are judiciously prescribed and carefully monitored, a polypharmacy approach can save lives. This is especially true when it comes to treating atherosclerosis. As you have learned, atherosclerosis is a complex disease that is influenced by a host of factors, including heredity, diet, exercise and stress. This is one of the reasons why understanding how to treat the disease has taken so long. But the fact that it is so complex has an upside. It gives us a lot of targets for treatment, from lowering LDL cholesterol to slowing blood clot formation.

When people take medications that attack atherosclerosis on a number of different fronts, their chances of surviving and maintaining good heart function greatly improve. The Scandinavian Simvastatin Survival Study that I mentioned earlier also demonstrated this. According to a review in the *Cleveland Clinic Journal of Medicine,* study participants with coronary artery disease were given a variety of treatments. Researchers found that those who were given no medications at all had a 29 per cent risk of dying or having a heart attack, stroke or some other major event within 5 years. Not very good odds. Those who were given statins had a much lower, 18.6 per cent, risk. Patients given a statin and aspirin had their risk lowered even more, to 11.2 per cent. The lucky ones were those who were given a statin, aspirin and a medication called a beta-blocker to lower blood pressure. Their risk of a major cardiac event was only 8.6 per cent. A later study showed that adding yet another drug, an ACE inhibitor, to this mix resulted in an even greater reduction. A review of this data published in the *Cleveland Clinic Journal of Medicine* estimated that the cumulative reduction would be 70 per cent.

The other advantage of polypharmacy therapy is the ability to keep the dosage of each medication below the level where it is likely to cause side effects. We did not always have this luxury. In my early days in training, we had a small fraction of the pharmaceutical choices we have today. We often had to push medications to the limit of toler-ance to control blood pressure or treat other problems. For example, beta-blockers were often prescribed at high dosages for the treatment of blood pressure, angina or abnormal heart rhythms. Patients were often extremely fatigued at the doses used. Today, we can take advan-tage of the therapeutic effects of beta-blockers but avoid their side effects by combining them with other medications.

I am well aware that taking multiple medications can be expen-sive. I also know that keeping so many prescriptions filled and remem-bering to take medications at the proper time can be annoying. But when the medications are medically necessary, the reward can be life itself.

Because taking multiple medications can have many benefits, two researchers from England and New Zealand made a bold proposal in the *British Medical Journal* in 2003. They suggested that a 'polypill' be created and recommended for everyone over the age of 55. This polypill would combine six generic heart medications, each one hav-ing been proven to reduce the risk of heart disease and stroke. Accord-ing to their calculations, 'The Polypill strategy, based on a single daily pill containing six components as specified, would prevent 88 per cent of heart attacks and 80 per cent of strokes. About 1 in 3 people would directly benefit, each, on average, gaining 11 to 12 years of life without a heart attack or stroke (20 years in those aged 55–64).' The researchers estimated that the polypill would save about 200,000 lives a year in Britain alone.

I don't think the polypill is such a bad idea, but I think we can do better by tailoring medications to each individual's risk profile.

It Can't Save Your Life If You Don't Take It

Almost daily, I find myself talking to a patient about the importance of taking the medications I recommend exactly as I have prescribed them. A few patients never fill their prescriptions. Others take their medications, but are eager to discontinue them because they have the understandable wish to be heart healthy and drug free.

Recently, I saw a new patient who was recovering from a heart attack. He told me that his previous doctor had put him on four different medications. 'He gave me a statin, two kinds of high blood pressure medications, and a blood thinner that's really a rat poison. Well, I stopped taking them all 2 months ago,' he said with a note of pride. 'And I feel better now than I did when I was taking them.' I explained to him that by stopping the medications, he was now right back to where he was before the heart attack.

While this scenario is common, a perhaps more troubling reason that people don't want to take heart medications is that they don't realize that atherosclerosis is a *chronic* condition. They think that once they've recovered from a heart attack or stroke or had bypass surgery or a stent put in, the underlying problem is gone. In a recent survey of heart attack victims, 41 per cent did not know that they were battling a lifelong problem. Nor did they understand that they had a very high risk of having another cardiac event. Without aggressive medical treatment, most people with atherosclerosis eventually die from it. But when patients are treated aggressively – and for many people that includes taking multiple medications – they have a good chance of living to a ripe old age.

I have had a few high-risk patients who were dead set against taking prescription medications of any kind, despite my best attempts to explain why I thought they were necessary. Scott was one of them. Scott had a strong family history of heart disease. His father, grandfather and two uncles had all died of heart problems before the age of 50. Scott was 53 years old when I first saw him, so he had managed to outlive all of his relatives by several years. This was undoubtedly because he was very conscientious about his diet and had been running 25 miles a week since his mid thirties.

To see if his health campaign was truly working, I ordered advanced blood tests and a CT scan. Unfortunately, the scan showed that his genes were carrying on the family tradition: despite his best efforts, he had a high Calcium Score for his age. The blood tests helped explain why his healthy habits had failed to protect him. First, he had high levels of lipoprotein (a), or Lp(a), an inherited risk factor that does not respond to diet or exercise. (As I discussed in Chapter 4, Lp(a) is the substance that helps LDL particles burrow into blood vessel walls, setting the stage for a heart attack.)

The second problem was that Scott's good HDL was only 1.1 mmol/L. Because he was an avid runner, it should have been 1.6 mmol/L or higher. This was another indication that his genes were defeating his best efforts. Finally, he also had high levels of C-reactive protein (CRP), another risk factor for heart disease (see pages 56–57). To lower these risk factors, I recommended that he take niacin to reduce the Lp(a) and that he also take a statin to reduce his LDL further and to reduce the inflammation indicated by the elevated CRP.

Scott refused to take the statin. He was determined to stay healthy through natural means alone. He agreed to try the niacin only because, as he put it, 'It isn't a drug.' I cautioned him that the niacin might cause skin flushes, a common reaction, but that they would diminish over time. He tried the niacin for a few days and then stopped taking it. 'I don't like the way it makes me feel,' he told me during his next visit.

I can advise my patients about what to do, but I can't make them comply. Ultimately, the course of Scott's treatment was up to him, and his choice was to go 'all natural'. I made one more plea. I cautioned, 'Given all that you're battling, the natural consequence of relying on all-natural remedies is a premature death.' He told me that

Andrew's Story

'My Calcium Score was over 1000!'

My mother had a heart attack at 43. She died from heart failure 2 years later. My dad's brother died from a heart attack at an early age, and my dad had a stroke when he was 63. I was really worried that something would happen to me, especially when I was 42 and 43. But when I turned 44, I lost some of the fear and did kind of a U-turn. I let my guard down for a few years and started eating and drinking whatever I wanted. I gained weight and my blood pressure went up. I was heading down the wrong road. That's when I read a magazine article about heart scans and decided to track Dr Agatston down.

The doctor did several tests, including a heart scan and a carotid ultrasound, and then gave me the results. There was good news and bad news. The good news was that my total cholesterol was 4.9 mmol/L. The bad news was that I had a bunch of plaque in all three of my major coronary arteries and the carotid arteries supplying my brain. I saw the actual images. I had a lot of plaque. My Calcium Score was over 1000! He told me the reason I had low total cholesterol but lots of plaque was that I had these small cholesterol particles that were just the right size to squeeze into my artery walls. It made sense. So, I had to accept the fact that, although I was only 46, I was a candidate for a heart attack or a stroke.

Dr Agatston told me that I needed aggressive drug therapy. I believed that drug therapy fuels the pharmacies of America, so I was resistant. I wanted to do it with diet alone. But I tell you, once you see a picture of your own heart and see all the plaque light up, you become a believer. My arteries looked like an airport runway at night, and on the scan, healthy arteries are supposed to look dark. So, I accepted the new game plan – diet, exercise and drugs.

I still bug Dr Agatston about allowing me to wean myself off the drugs. But he says that as long as I tolerate my medications and there is no sign of increasing plaque, he wants me to stay on the programme. He reminded me that the goal was to keep me alive, not get me off medications. I keep seeing the picture of my clogged arteries, and I totally agree. ∎

he would be even more careful about what he ate and run 40 miles a week. He was going to be so fit that death couldn't catch him.

I was concerned but not surprised when I got a call from Mount Sinai Hospital about 2 years later informing me that Scott had been admitted to Accident and Emergency. He had been jogging over the Rickenbacker Causeway from Miami to Key Biscayne when he experienced chest pains. He was taken to hospital and diagnosed with unstable angina, a sign that a heart attack could be imminent. Later that day, he underwent angioplasty. The good news was that he hadn't suffered an actual heart attack. His was a classic example of acute coronary syndrome in which a plaque rupture caused severe chest pain but not a heart attack itself. Scott was one of those lucky people who receive a warning signal before a heart attack occurs.

The scare convinced Scott that he really did need to take medications to overcome his bad genes. Today, he takes niacin along with a statin, and I am pleased to report that he continues his healthy lifestyle habits. Chances are good that he will be the first male in his family for several generations to experience old age. Much of the credit goes to him for his own efforts, but credit is also owed to the heart medications that are taking care of the risk factors he cannot change. When a healthy lifestyle is combined with state-of-the-art diagnosis and appropriate medications, even a strong family history of heart disease can be overcome.

8

IS THIS PROCEDURE
REALLY NECESSARY?

Two crucial questions must be answered when considering whether
an invasive approach to treating heart disease is necessary.

First, you must ask, *Will this procedure prolong my life?* If the procedure is likely to prevent a heart attack in the future or stop one in its
tracks, thereby saving heart muscle, then the procedure is clearly indicated to prolong your life.

If the answer to the first question is 'No', then you must also ask,
Will this procedure improve my quality of life? Certainly if you are experiencing significant chest pain or discomfort or other heart-related
symptoms that occur with normal daily activities, the pain has already
affected your quality of life and an invasive procedure is usually desirable. If you are athletic and chest pain is interfering with your ability
to exercise as vigorously as usual, then you may want to consider having an invasive procedure to relieve the pain, even if it will not clearly
prolong your life.

The four-step prevention programme described in Part 2 of this
book (and that I prescribe every day in my practice) is intended to
keep my patients from ever reaching the point of needing an invasive
procedure. But if you are already there because of too little prevention
too late, invasive action may be required and possibly lifesaving.
Sometimes, however, chest pain from a coronary blockage can be
reversed and exercise capacity improved with medication and lifestyle
changes alone. This chapter will help you work with your doctor to
make your decision if an invasive procedure is being considered.

Invasive Procedures

To better understand when an invasive procedure is essential and when it may not be needed, you first need a bit of background on what an angiogram, angioplasty and bypass involve.

Invasive Angiogram

The invasive angiogram was once considered the 'gold standard' for diagnosing atherosclerosis. It is still the best method of assessing the *per cent blockage* of a coronary artery, but as we have discussed, there is a lot more to evaluating heart disease than just per cent blockage. Too often, there is a tendency to 'treat the angiogram' rather than the patient. This leads to the unnecessary opening of areas of partial blockage that are not significantly compromising bloodflow and are not at risk for future plaque rupture and heart attack.

How is it done? In an invasive angiogram, a cardiologist inserts a catheter into an artery, typically in the groin area (but occasionally in the arm). The catheter is threaded through the femoral artery and up through the aorta until it reaches the coronary arteries located where the aorta arises from the left ventricle (the main pumping chamber of the heart). A dye is injected through the catheter into the coronary arteries and x-ray images are recorded. The resulting pictures show the width of the inside of the coronary arteries where blood is flowing (this area is called the *lumen*). If there is a narrowing of the diameter of the vessel, it is measured to determine the amount of blockage. (The angiogram does not show plaque embedded inside the vessel walls, however.) Depending on what is found, angioplasty or bypass surgery may be recommended to restore bloodflow.

Angioplasty

Since it was first performed in 1977, angioplasty has been considered the less invasive alternative to bypass surgery. Angioplasty is done to relieve chest pain by opening the offending obstruction that is compromising bloodflow to a significant amount of heart muscle. When chest pain is present and a large amount of muscle is compromised (this must be determined by a cardiologist), then the consensus of opinion is that opening the offending vessel with angioplasty is a good idea. If a small area of muscle is affected, then prescribing lifestyle changes and medications is usually appropriate. In cases where a patient wants to be pain free but doesn't want to wait for lifestyle changes to have an effect, angioplasty may still be appropriate. But remember, the overwhelming evidence is that opening a chronic obstruction to relieve pain *will not* prevent a future heart attack or prolong life.

How does the success rate for angioplasty compare to an aggressive programme of cholesterol-lowering medications when dealing with chronic blockages? In a famous study known as the AVERT trial, patients with mild to moderate coronary artery disease were either given a maximum dose of the statin drug atorvastatin (Lipitor) to drive down their cholesterol or received angioplasty and medication (which could include a statin) at the discretion of their doctor. When the results were reported in the *New England Journal of Medicine* in 1999, cardiologists were surprised to learn that the patients taking the high-dose statin drugs fared better than those who had undergone angioplasty. The drug-treated patients required fewer hospitalizations, subsequent angioplasties and bypass surgeries than the angioplasty group.

The evidence against the use of angioplasty to prevent heart attack in those with chronic heart disease is strong. In 2005, the American Heart Association journal *Circulation* published an analysis of several studies comparing angioplasty versus medical therapy. They reviewed a total of 2950 cardiac patients. Of these, 1476 received angioplasty and 1474 received noninvasive treatment, such as drug therapy and dietary intervention. The finding: compared with conservative medical treatment, angioplasty did not decrease mortality or the risk of heart attack during follow-up in patients with chronic coronary artery disease.

How is it done? During angioplasty, a catheter is threaded into a coronary artery in the same manner as described for an angiogram. However, it is advanced through the affected artery to the area of the blockage to be opened. Next, a balloon-tipped wire is threaded into the catheter and positioned in the middle of the blockage. The balloon is inflated to compress the plaque against the artery wall and enlarge the artery opening. The balloon is then removed, and the plaque is typically held in place with a wire mesh tube called a *stent*. While circulation to the heart is usually restored, the presence of the stent does not prevent plaque from developing elsewhere in the same artery or in other coronary arteries.

Bypass Surgery

The official name is *coronary artery bypass grafting*, or CABG, but most people simply call it *bypass surgery*. While bypass surgery was truly a breakthrough in the treatment of heart disease, its ability to prolong life as opposed to relieving chest pain has been called into question by studies comparing it to a noninvasive medical approach.

How is it done? In this procedure, after the patient is anaesthetized, the surgeon 'cracks the chest', an irreverent phrase used to refer to the process of sawing through a patient's sternum (breastbone) and opening the chest cavity with spreaders. Next, the patient is put on a heart-lung machine so that the heart can be stilled during the critical part of the surgery. (More recently, some surgeons are performing 'off pump' bypass on the beating heart.)

Once the patient is prepared, a vein the diameter of a drinking straw is generally 'harvested' from another part of the body, usually the leg. One end of the vein is attached to the aorta (the primary blood vessel leading from the heart to the body), and the other end is attached to the artery beyond the site of the blockage.

Another way to bypass a blockage is by using arteries in your chest called *internal mammary arteries*. Radial arteries from your arm may also be used. Whenever it is technically feasible, arterial bypasses are favoured over those done with veins because they are much less likely to become clogged themselves.

Exciting advances are now being made in performing minimally invasive (including robotic) bypass surgery.

I f your doctor says you need *nonemergency* angioplasty or bypass surgery and you do not feel that you have significant symptoms, I recommend that you seek a second opinion from a cardiologist who specializes in prevention, not procedures. Call your local teaching hospital or a major medical centre and ask for a referral to a nonintervental cardiologist, preferably one with an interest in preventive cardiology. A doctor who practises prevention will bring a different perspective to your case and may have ideas about noninvasive treatment.

Complications

Each of the procedures covered on the previous pages can have complications, including heart attack or stroke. While these complications are rare with a nonemergency angiogram and uncommon with elective angioplasty, they are much more likely to occur with bypass surgery. Furthermore, bypass surgery can produce decreased cognitive function and sometimes dementia in certain people, a complication that I feel is underestimated.

Naturally, with any of these procedures, the more experienced the cardiologist or surgeon, the better the results. Complication rates can vary widely depending on the severity of a person's illness and the skill of the practitioner. Before you undergo any invasive procedure, be sure to thoroughly discuss the possibility of complications with your cardiologist and surgeon.

Stories from My Practice

Now that you know more about how these procedures are performed, let's take a look at some patient case histories. I have organized them by symptom, from no symptoms to acute, to help put invasive cardiology into perspective. The patients' names have been changed as have some of the details. You may recognize yourself in one of them. If you do, I hope you will take immediate action and discuss any symptoms you may be having with your doctor.

What If You Have No Symptoms or Atypical Symptoms?

The first goal of preventive cardiology should be to treat risk factors early enough that an invasive procedure is never needed. Another important goal, however, is to decrease the number of bypass surgeries and angioplasties being performed on those with 'no' symptoms or 'atypical' symptoms.

'No' symptoms literally means that you have no chest discomfort, shortness of breath, or other heart-related symptoms when you are at rest or during exertion. Keep in mind, though, that in some people, the heart has the ability to produce a network of collateral blood vessels (see page 29). In such cases, a person could have the three major coronary arteries largely blocked and still have no symptoms. That's why getting a heart scan and the advanced blood testing I describe in Step 3 is so important.

'Atypical' symptoms are chest pains or other symptoms that do not indicate a limitation of bloodflow through your coronary arteries. For example, fleeting, sharp chest pains that last just seconds and occur at rest but not with exertion are not characteristic of inadequate bloodflow to your heart. As I describe on page 200, there are features of shortness of breath that strongly indicate they are not from significant heart or lung disease. That said, only your doctor can determine whether a chest pain is typical or atypical, so never try to diagnose any new chest pain, fleeting or not, by yourself.

Let me tell you the stories of Richard, Rita, Josh and Joe.

SHOULD I HAVE IT?

Recently, I received a message from my friend Richard, who lives in New York City. His doctor had urged him to have an angiogram as soon as possible, and Richard wanted my advice. I immediately returned his call, thinking that Richard must be lying in a hospital coronary care unit somewhere, in pain and attached to an IV. Imagine my surprise when his wife told me that he wasn't at home or in the hospital, but on the tennis court – playing. 'Hmm, I guess this angiogram might not be so urgent,' I thought.

When I spoke to Richard later, he reported that during a routine checkup, his doctor had recommended a heart scan (the 64-slice CT noninvasive angiogram) to see if he had any coronary artery blockages. Richard had agreed to have the procedure. After the heart scan, the doctor told him that he did, in fact, have what looked like a blockage of one of his coronary arteries and that he should have an invasive angiogram performed to get a definitive diagnosis. Richard told me that the doctor was really pushing for the invasive angiogram. 'What should I do?' he asked me. 'Should I have it?'

Knowing that Richard had just been out playing tennis, I suspected the answer was going to be 'No!' But I wanted to make sure, so I gathered some more information. I cross-examined him. 'How are you feeling? How is your exercise capacity? Have you had any chest pain? Any undue shortness of breath?' His answers: 'I feel great. I played an hour of singles, no problem. I've had no chest pain or shortness of breath. Nothing's different than usual.' But Richard was still worried. The very next day he hopped on a plane to Miami with his heart scan images in hand.

At my office, I gave Richard a nuclear exercise stress test, and he practically burned up the treadmill. (The test, which I explain on pages 212–14, determines if the bloodflow through your coronary arteries can increase enough to adequately supply your hardworking heart muscle.) In Richard's case, the stress test indicated that he had excellent exercise capacity compared to most people and that he was in especially fine shape for a 69-year-old. He had no chest discomfort or undue shortness of breath, and the bloodflow to his heart muscle was absolutely normal, even during the hardest part of the test.

When I reviewed Richard's heart scan, it was debatable whether or not he actually had a blockage. But even if he did, opening or bypassing it could not improve symptoms that didn't exist in the first place. Nor would such a procedure decrease his risk of a heart attack.

Since bypass surgery or angioplasty was, in my opinion, unnecessary, there was no reason for Richard to undergo an invasive angiogram. Richard's answers to the two questions I ask everyone to think about would have to be 'No' and 'No'.

NOT SO LUCKY

Another all-too-common scenario is illustrated by the story of Rita, a 60-year-old who underwent a nuclear exercise stress test with her own doctor because she was experiencing fleeting, nonexertional pains in her chest. Rita did not have these pains during her daily workout or when feeling particularly stressed, but felt them at unpredictable times.

During the stress test, she demonstrated very good exercise capacity and experienced no chest discomfort. Her electrocardiogram, or ECG (which measures the electrical activity of the heart), remained normal during the test. However, her nuclear images from the test showed evidence of a possible blockage.

Rita's doctor sent her to have an invasive angiogram, which revealed a 65 per cent narrowing of her left anterior descending coronary artery. An angioplasty was performed to open it, and Rita was told that she was lucky to have had the procedure because it likely averted a heart attack.

Initially Rita felt fine (as she had before the procedure). But then, 2 months later, she began to experience chest tightness during her daily jog, which disappeared when she stopped running. She had never experienced chest discomfort during her jog before. Her doctor said he would need to do another angiogram to check the site of the angioplasty.

Unfortunately, the artery in which the angioplasty had been performed was now 80 per cent blocked due to restenosis, a common complication of this procedure. Restenosis occurs when the site of the crushed plaque heals with a large scar that limits bloodflow. Rita underwent another angioplasty to restore the good circulation that had been present before her first procedure.

Rita was not as lucky as Richard. While she had complained of fleeting chest pains, a doctor should have known that they were clearly not from her heart. So what should the answers to the two questions have been in Rita's case? Remember, Rita's excellent exercise capacity could not have been improved by either angioplasty or bypass surgery. And because her heart function was normal, neither angioplasty nor a bypass would improve her longevity. *So the answers to both questions for Rita, had they been asked, would have been 'No'.* In fact, her first angioplasty was never necessary.

Case histories like Richard's and Rita's are common. I am often asked for a second opinion by patients who have had invasive approaches recommended when they have no symptoms or who have atypical symptoms that aren't due to a blockage. *The research is absolutely clear that in patients with no or atypical symptoms and good exercise capacity and good heart function, there is no need for either angioplasty or bypass surgery.*

A CALCIUM SCORE OF MORE THAN 500

Let me tell you about another patient, Josh, whom I have now followed for many years. When Josh was in his late fifties, he went for a heart scan and found out that he had a Calcium Score of more than 500, very high for his age. He underwent an exercise stress test that demonstrated excellent exercise capacity: he had no chest pain and no reduction of coronary bloodflow. This was consistent with the fact that he exercised regularly and fairly vigorously.

Although Josh was reassured by his doctor that he could be treated without an invasive procedure, he was and is a bit of a hypochondriac. For this reason, he insisted on an angiogram to really make sure everything was all right. His doctor agreed. The finding: three vessels were blocked more than 75 per cent. Although Josh's heart function was normal, as seen from the stress test, he underwent triple bypass surgery nevertheless.

When Josh moved to South Florida a year after his surgery and came to see me, I took his medical history and discussed the surgery. It wasn't until I got to know him better (and I had educated him on the basics of the plumbing-versus-healing model of heart disease) that he volunteered, 'Doc, I didn't need that surgery, did I?' My answer was 'No, Josh, you didn't.' I explained that, given his prior good exercise capacity and excellent exercise test results, adequate bloodflow was clearly reaching his heart muscle. For this to happen, he must have developed his own network of blood vessels to bypass the blockages (the *collateral circulation* I described earlier). Often these collateral vessels are too small to be seen on an angiogram, which is why Josh's doctor hadn't known about them.

I told Josh that bypass surgery is indicated in three clear situations. First, if lifestyle-limiting angina (chest pain) is present and cannot be improved with lifestyle changes, medications or angioplasty. Second, when the *left main coronary artery*, the very origin of the heart's circulatory system, is significantly obstructed. And third, when angina is present *and* there is a significant decrease in the function of the main pumping chamber of the heart (the left ventricle) *and* it is apparent that the left circumflex artery, the left anterior descending artery, and the right coronary artery all have blockages. Josh didn't fit any of the three criteria, even with the blockages (remember, he didn't have chest pain), so in his case, surgery would neither prolong his life nor improve his quality of life.

Fortunately, Josh survived his surgery without major complications and has continued to do well on an aggressive prevention programme. I feel badly that it was his initial heart scan that started him down the slippery slope to invasive interventions. This was an inappropriate use of the scan. But his heart scan did correctly indicate that he had extensive atherosclerosis and was at high risk for a heart attack. This was certainly confirmed by his angiogram. The lesson is that after the stress test showed excellent bloodflow to his heart and normal heart function, there was no need to go further. He should simply have been put on preventive lifestyle measures and treated aggressively with medications at that point.

UNEXPECTED COMPLICATIONS

Unfortunately, another patient who underwent bypass surgery did not ultimately fare as well as Josh. This was Joe, who first visited a cardiologist because he had become alarmed by a high blood pressure reading at his doctor's surgery. Joe had no chest pain or other symptoms, and at the age of 65 he continued to work and exercise vigorously. His doctor administered a nuclear exercise stress test. Although his exercise capacity was excellent, there was a question about a small compromise in bloodflow. Joe then had an angiogram, which showed three blockages of more than 70 per cent.

As with Josh, Joe's heart function was good, yet he too underwent bypass surgery. The big difference was that Joe's postoperative recovery was complicated by heart rhythm problems that required many doctor visits over several months. Eventually the heart rhythm problems resolved, but they wouldn't be Joe's biggest problem. After the surgery, he never seemed to be quite the same man he had been before the bypass. As it turned out, he was developing progressive dementia, which ended up shortening the length of his life and ruining its quality. As I mentioned earlier, decreased cognitive function and even dementia are known complications of bypass surgery, although the number of people who experience these problems is hard to quantify. Nevertheless, these complications are concerns that should be factored in when surgery is suggested for anyone, especially someone with nonexistent or atypical symptoms and a good quality of life.

What If You Have Mild Chronic Symptoms?

Mild chronic symptoms are chest discomfort (angina), shortness of breath, or other heart-related symptoms that occur fairly predictably with significant exertion or other stress. These symptoms might occur when you're carrying a heavy briefcase through an airport while rushing to catch a plane. Or they might occur while you're sprinting for a ball during a tennis game. The overall symptom pattern will be consistent, usually over a period of weeks or months or even over years (if ignored).

In the case of mild symptoms, there is more wiggle room to make a case for an invasive approach. But here again, it is important to answer the same two questions: *Will an invasive approach prolong my life?* and *Will an invasive approach improve my quality of life?* Again, let's look at some real-life case histories.

A BIG MISTAKE

Carol was a 62-year-old college professor when she had a heart scan that indicated a high Calcium Score. She had chosen not to take a statin because of a concern that it might affect her liver. Her diet was rather poor and her exercise regime was inconsistent at best.

While visiting New York to attend a winter academic conference, Carol decided to go jogging in Central Park. After running for 10 minutes, she noticed tightness and pain in the centre of her chest. Both symptoms went away when she rested but recurred the next day with similar exertion in the chilly weather. She thought right away that it might be angina, but she returned to Miami and did not report her experience to her doctor. This was a mistake. As I've said before, a person with chest pain should *always* call his or her doctor to discuss it.

Because of her concern, Carol decided to go on the South Beach Diet and began regular treadmill exercise. She lost about 14 kg (30 lb), became much fitter, and felt better than ever. The following summer, during her annual physical, she told her doctor about the episodes in New York the previous winter. He performed a nuclear exercise stress test to evaluate her prior symptoms. During the test, Carol demonstrated her new and improved exercise capacity, but she also admitted to the slightest chest tightness when she was 'running uphill' at the end of the stress test. Her nuclear images indicated some compromise in bloodflow, though her heart function was normal.

An angiogram was ordered and three blocked vessels were found. Bypass surgery was performed with some nearly lethal complications, but fortunately Carol survived. She is now on heart-protective medications and is doing very well.

But was her surgery necessary? First, was it likely to prolong her life? The answer is 'No'. Her heart function was already good, and her exercise capacity was already excellent. Second, was the surgery needed to improve her lifestyle? Again, the answer is 'No'. She had never had any problem with her daily exercise routine or with any other activities. It is likely that by simply treating Carol with the preventive measures she had already adopted, plus the heart-protective medications she ended up taking after the surgery, her symptoms would have resolved on their own and the surgery could have been avoided.

OVERCOMING BAD GENES

Another case to consider is that of Kevin, who was 55 when he came to me with rather mild symptoms. He was one of those patients who, because of a family history of heart disease, had adopted a healthy lifestyle a few years earlier in an attempt to overcome his bad genes. This included taking up competitive running and participating in several marathons after he had turned 50.

During his training, Kevin had noticed chest pressure, usually occurring only after he had run several miles and often when he was running uphill. It was relieved when he slowed down and reached a flat surface. This pain had recurred over a month.

Although Kevin had learned several years before experiencing any symptoms that he had a high Calcium Score and a slightly elevated level of bad LDL cholesterol, he had been unwilling to take a medication to lower his cholesterol. Furthermore, his good HDL was at the lower limit of normal – not what you would expect in a marathoner (the HDLs of long-distance runners are usually off the charts). He didn't want to deal with that either.

I was almost certain that Kevin's pain was angina caused by a blockage in one of his coronary arteries. An ECG and the nuclear images from a stress test confirmed this. Even so, his exercise capacity was excellent.

What should be done? Would opening his obstruction prolong his life? Based on the outcomes of well-regarded angioplasty studies, the answer was 'No'. But Kevin was a special case. The studies on angioplasty did not include a large number of marathoners who might be dehydrated and totally exhausted at the end of a race – two factors that can predispose a runner to a heart attack. Would an angioplasty improve his quality of life? Here the answer was 'Yes'. Whether or not Kevin ever entered another marathon, exercise was essential to his enjoyment of daily life. What's more, he and I were convinced that his exercise regime had helped him to partially overcome his bad family genes. It was really important that he keep it up.

Kevin did undergo an angiogram, and an 80 per cent obstruction was found, opened and stented in his left anterior descending coronary artery. Today he has returned to his running and has agreed to take medications to help overcome his bad genes. Now pushing 60, he continues to do well, and I expect his good health and excellent quality of life to continue. Kevin is an example of a situation where mild symptoms did, in my opinion, warrant an invasive solution.

There is one additional point I'd like to make here about stress and exercise. I advise my patients with already existing coronary artery disease, as well as those at risk, not to take on vigorous or competitive exercise if they are not in shape for it. Competitive situations, whether at a company picnic or on the tennis court or football pitch, can often seduce the underconditioned to push a bit too hard. Do you recognize yourself?

The problem with these situations is that they cause very large pulses of adrenaline to be released into the bloodstream. This can cause an otherwise harmless plaque rupture to turn into a heart attack. Kevin was a trained athlete, and his regular exercise sessions would not cause the same adrenaline rush that would occur if an untrained individual tried to keep up with him during a run. It is not the exercise that is bad. Regular exercise is crucial for good health. It is the sudden change in activity level that can cause trouble. *Moral:* Talk to your doctor before starting any kind of exercise programme, and don't perform levels of exercise that you aren't trained for.

What If You Have Moderate to Severe Symptoms?

Moderate heart-related symptoms are those that occur as you're going about the normal activities of daily life or with just a little exertion. In contrast to the mild chest pains (angina) described earlier, these symptoms tend to occur while you're simply walking through an airport without bags or during the normal course of a tennis game, when you're not even running hard for a ball. Severe symptoms mean that the chest pains occur with even less exertion or stress. Let's look at Roger as an example of someone with severe symptoms.

A MISLEADING TEST

One day, I thought I was seeing a new patient who would be routine. Roger was a 55-year-old male who had been on a statin for 7 years because of an elevated cholesterol level. Normally he did spinning classes several days a week at the gym for exercise, but he had decreased his regular routine over the busy December holiday season. In January, when he started spinning again, he noticed chest discomfort with 'not so much' exercise.

As it happened, he'd had an exercise stress test the previous November that had been normal. So when he called his doctor in January to tell him about his discomfort, the doctor said he wasn't concerned because of that excellent test.

Roger came to see me in February and said he was experiencing chest discomfort when simply walking from the lift to my office. He had not exercised since his attempt in January because of these symptoms. In fact, his symptoms at this time were so indicative of a significant blockage that I sent him straight to the cath lab for an angiogram.

Roger's angiogram showed significant obstruction of his left main coronary artery as well as greater than 70 per cent blockages of his three major coronary arteries.

What was the next step? Would bypass surgery or angioplasty prolong his life? The answer: a resounding 'Yes' for surgery. As I mentioned earlier, obstruction of the left main coronary artery is a clear indication for a bypass. While this decision was already made in order to save his life, what about the second question? Would an invasive approach make a difference in Roger's quality of life? This was also an easy answer. Roger had been miserable and unable to do his usual activities for nearly 2 months. Surgery would clearly help.

It's been 5 years since Roger's surgery, and he's doing very well. But there are a few more lessons to be learned from his case. First, when I did a baseline heart scan (see pages 208–10) on Roger after his surgery, it showed a Calcium Score of well over 1000. Therefore, it was clear to me that the extent of his problem could have been determined much earlier, before he had symptoms, *if* he had been given the scan earlier (I recommend one for most men beginning at the age of 40).

Second, though Roger's LDL cholesterol had been well controlled with a statin for 7 years and his lifestyle was admirable, he still continued to accumulate plaque until an apparent plaque rupture caused his first symptoms. Again, this could have been predicted much earlier with advanced blood testing and a heart scan. When I finally did get the results of an advanced blood test, much too late to prevent the surgery, it showed me that Roger's HDL was low and his HDL particle size was quite small. He was a heart attack waiting to happen.

Today Roger takes prescription niacin, and his total HDL and his HDL particle size have improved dramatically. Roger's was a situation where a combination of medications had to be added to lifestyle changes to overcome his bad genes. And I anticipate that Roger will lead a long and very enjoyable life.

What If Your Symptoms Are Acute?

There are times when an invasive approach is instantly appropriate, necessary and even lifesaving. When a patient experiences the rapid onset of chest discomfort *and* the pains last for several minutes *and* your doctor determines it is likely due to a blockage, then the prompt performance of an angiogram is essential to find the 'culprit' plaque that is responsible. This is typically followed by restoration of blood-flow by opening the artery with angioplasty or, occasionally, by bypassing it with emergency surgery. The decision to perform an invasive procedure must be made by a cardiologist. Of course, a percentage of angiograms will turn out to be normal, but the risk of the procedure is worth it if a heart attack can be stopped in its tracks.

An alternative to directly opening an acute blockage is to use a clot-busting medication such as a tissue plasminogen activator (tPA). This is commonly used in hospitals that do not have emergency cath labs on the premises. While not quite as effective, it is a good alternative to angioplasty or bypass and can dissolve the offending blood clot.

It is very important that men and women with new, and especially persistent, episodes of chest discomfort immediately seek medical help. There may be false alarms, but calling the doctor is critical in order to interrupt a potentially deadly or damaging heart attack. If you think you are experiencing a heart attack, time is of the essence. The following are two cases in point:

IT WASN'T INDIGESTION

Recently, I was told of the sudden death of a young practising doctor who succumbed to a heart attack at home. It was later that I learned he had experienced waxing and waning chest pains during the week prior to his death. He was apparently treating himself with antacids in the mistaken belief that he was experiencing indigestion. Clearly, soft plaque had ruptured and, as is typical of an acute coronary syndrome, the clot kept reforming and dissolving until ultimately it grew and completely blocked one of his major coronary arteries. This is what led to his tragic, preventable death. I also learned that this doctor had a family history of heart disease but had never taken the time to have a good cardiac workup. Tragic!

A HAPPY ENDING

A happier ending resulted for my friend Thomas, who had sold his company and retired at the age of 65. To make sure he would enjoy a healthy retirement, Thomas underwent a cardiac workup including an exercise stress test just prior to moving to South Florida. He was told that he passed with flying colours and had the heart of a 50-year-old.

Armed with this knowledge, Thomas couldn't believe that the chest pain and tightness he suddenly experienced while doing moderate treadmill exercise a couple of weeks after his stress test could possibly be from his heart. Nevertheless, he stopped exercising, went home and rested.

Having had no further pain at home, Thomas returned to the treadmill the next day and experienced the same feelings. But this time they occurred with only light exercise. And, unlike the day before, the pain was accompanied by a cold sweat and weakness.

Thomas was now really alarmed and told a fellow exerciser who happened to be a doctor what was going on. The doctor called an ambulance and me immediately. While I waited for Thomas to arrive at the hospital, I notified the cath lab to be ready for a coronary emergency. Upon arrival, an ECG clearly indicated that Thomas was indeed having a heart attack. In the cath lab, an acute blockage in his right coronary artery was successfully opened with angioplasty, quickly restoring bloodflow to his heart muscle. Thomas's resulting heart damage was minimal and he returned to an active, healthy and happy retirement. Ten years later, with an aggressive prevention programme, including plenty of exercise, a good diet and medications, I am pleased to report that Thomas is doing fine.

Take Action!

I hope in recounting all of these stories that I have convinced you that any new onset of chest discomfort must be taken seriously and acted upon promptly. Remember that even if the pain goes away spontaneously, it does not mean you are in the clear. It is not the time to ask for a second opinion.

PART

2

THE
SOUTH
BEACH
HEART
PROGRAMME

In Part 1 of this book, you learned that we have the tools to prevent most heart attacks and strokes. Living without heart disease is within our reach. And more to the point, it's within *your* reach. Now, in Part 2, you will get a blueprint for aggressively preventing heart disease on your own and with the help of your doctor. The South Beach Heart Programme is the four-step prevention plan that I employ every day in my cardiology practice.

STEP 1
Following the Principles
of the South Beach Diet

The first step in heart disease prevention is good nutrition. Eating the right foods can help you maintain a healthy weight; improve your cholesterol, triglycerides and other blood fats; lower your blood pressure; and help to keep you heart attack free. This step is based on the healthy eating principles of the South Beach Diet, an eating plan that has helped my cardiac and diabetes patients for more than 10 years. If you're already on the South Beach Diet, you're doing a lot to keep your cardiovascular system in good condition. If you're new to the diet, a special section, 'The South Beach Diet: A Crash Course' (see pages 146–64) will get you started right away.

STEP 2
The South Beach Heart Workout

The second step of the programme provides a comprehensive but simple workout that stretches and strengthens your muscles, burns fat and improves your cardiovascular system. It takes advantage of the latest knowledge on how to exercise safely and effectively. You will learn the importance of a core, functional approach to conditioning and why and how many of us have become deconditioned. Again and again, medical research has shown that people who eat well and exercise regularly have a lower risk of virtually all diseases, including heart disease. If you've never engaged in a regular exercise programme before, Step 2 will show you how easy it is to incorporate fitness into your life. If you work out already, Step 2 will help you maximize the beneficial effects of your efforts.

STEP 3
Getting the Right Diagnostic Tests

The right diagnostic tests – heart imaging, advanced blood testing and more – can detect heart disease in its earliest stages, when it can still be slowed or reversed. The earlier you get these tests, the better your chances of preventing a heart attack or stroke. Of course, a test won't do you any good if you don't get it. Step 3 explains how to work with your doctor to obtain these diagnostic tests, when and how often to get them, what each test is like and what the results can tell you.

STEP 4
Getting the Right Medications

Today we have effective medications to improve bad cholesterol, increase good cholesterol, reduce blood pressure and control a number of other risk factors for heart disease. The problem is, these medications are often underprescribed, or when they are prescribed, they're not taken because patients do not sufficiently understand their benefits. To give you a striking statistic: only about 50 per cent of people at high risk for heart disease who could benefit from taking a cholesterol-lowering medicine are actually receiving one. If more people who needed these state-of-the-art medications actually got them, we would do much better at preventing heart attacks and strokes. Furthermore, it would drastically reduce the number of angioplasties and bypass surgeries that are being performed in this country. Step 4 of this prevention programme is about making sure that you have the latest information on medications. I urge you to work with your doctor to take advantage of the incredible advances that have occurred in this area of medicine over the past two decades.

· · · · · · ·

Remember, each step of the South Beach Heart Programme is important. If you have risk factors for heart disease, you should work with your doctor to get advanced blood tests, heart imaging and the medications that you may need. You can easily get started with the first two steps of the programme on your own. If you already have a good relationship with a doctor, I urge you to have a discussion with him or her about what you've learned from this book. If you don't have good communication with your doctor, I suggest that you ask for a second opinion, ideally with a prevention-oriented doctor or cardiologist.

STEP

1

FOLLOWING THE PRINCIPLES OF THE SOUTH BEACH DIET

Although I am a cardiologist, not a diet doctor, with nearly 30 years of medical experience in performing diagnostic tests and prescribing medications, my first recommendation for preventing heart disease is to lead a healthy lifestyle. The foundation of healthy living is a sound diet and regular exercise. That's why Step 1 of my prevention programme encourages you to follow the heart-healthy eating principles of the South Beach Diet and Step 2 shows you how to incorporate exercise into your everyday life. Both are complementary and both are essential for optimal cardiac health.

From my experience with patients and friends, I have found that when you eat well, you exercise better, and vice versa. For one thing, eating a healthy diet gives you the energy to exercise. And exercise burns calories, increases insulin sensitivity, and produces feel-good endorphins, which all contribute to healthy weight management.

I developed the South Beach Diet more than 10 years ago primarily for my existing heart patients and for those with elevated cholesterol, prediabetes, diabetes and high blood pressure who were at high risk for heart disease. By following its healthy eating principles, you too can reduce your risk of heart attack and stroke.

If you're already familiar with the South Beach Diet, this chapter gives you additional information on how it can specifically help your heart. For those of you who are new to the diet, you should know that it is far more than a weight-loss programme. Good nutrition is the cornerstone of a healthy heart and a healthy body. You can't have one without the other. When you consistently eat the right carbohydrates (nutrient-dense, fibre-rich vegetables, whole fruits and whole grains), lean protein, low-fat dairy and the right fats, you give your body the nutrients it needs to help regulate your blood pressure, fight cell-damaging inflammation, establish normal cholesterol and triglyceride levels, and reduce the risk of potentially deadly blood clots.

These principles are based on the way we were designed to eat. The obesity, diabetes and heart disease epidemics of the Western world reflect the degree to which we have strayed from our nutritional heritage. If we can integrate healthy eating and exercise into our busy lives, we can dramatically change the health of our nation.

I go into more detail about the basic principles of the South Beach Diet – and how you can make it a way of life – on pages 146–64. But first, some background.

Changing the Way People Eat

The success of the original South Beach Diet book has given me a unique opportunity to help change the way people eat – and this has become an important goal for me. Today, many Westerners, particularly Americans, have horrible eating habits. Between our busy lifestyles and the availability of fast food on practically every street corner, we're killing ourselves with our consumption of high-fat burgers and sugary milkshakes, trans fat-laden fried foods, highly refined foods with minimal nutrient value, and other unhealthy food choices. Our plates are full of bad fats and bad carbs and stripped of the heart-healthy, fibre-rich fruits, vegetables and whole grains that are so important to maintaining good health.

If we had deliberately set out to design a diet to make people fat, diabetic and candidates for premature death from heart attack or stroke, we couldn't have done a better job. Furthermore, until recently, we received confusing, conflicting and often wrong information from governments and from nutritional experts about what constitutes a healthy diet. Thankfully, that is changing.

The Diet Debates Are Over

Today, the diet debates are over. We have moved beyond the confusion of the low-fat versus low-carb battles to an expert consensus on what constitutes a healthy diet. Health-care professionals now agree that our focus should be on nutrient-dense, fibre-rich carbohydrates, healthy sources of unsaturated fats, low-fat dairy and lean sources of protein. Undoubtedly, ongoing research will continue to add a great deal to our knowledge of the benefits of individual foods, but the basic principles of healthy eating are not going to change.

To better understand how we got into the health mess we are in and how we have come to the present consensus of opinion, it's important to be aware of some relevant history.

When I began work on the South Beach Diet, the only other diets recommended for heart patients in the US were either the standard low-fat, low-calorie eating plan endorsed by the American Heart Association or the even stricter, extremely low-fat regimes popularized by Dr Dean Ornish and Nathan Pritikin. At the time, telling patients to eat fat of any sort was medical heresy.

The premise of the low-fat diet was simple. Experts believed that the American diet was too high in fat. They based their belief, in part, on a major study published in the 1970s that compared a society's diet to its rate of heart disease. The study, which was conducted by a brilliant researcher named Ancel Keys, PhD, of the University of Minnesota, identified a direct correlation between fat intake and heart attack.

Dr Keys's study found that residents of the United States and certain countries in Europe had both the highest intake of total fat and the highest rate of heart attack. Countries with lower fat intake had much lower rates of heart disease. It was well known that people in less developed countries with very low fat intakes had almost no heart attacks.

The study identified one exception to the rule. In Crete, people ate a relatively high-fat diet but still had low rates of heart disease. Since the results for Crete were not consistent with the rest of the study, they were discounted. What the researchers did not appreciate at that time was that, although the typical Crete diet was high in fat, the fat was 'good' fat from olive oil, oily fish and nuts, not the bad saturated fat that was consumed in the countries whose populations had the highest rates of heart attack. What they also didn't understand was the fact that people who lived in countries that consumed the least amount of fat also ate the highest amount of *fibre*, which we now know is protective against heart disease. In fact, in 1980, when Dr Keys wrote a book summarizing his research, he suggested that fibre may have been an important variable not taken into account at the time of his study. This was not an oversight, because the role of fibre in nutrition was not known at the time of his study.

But the initial response of the medical community to Dr Keys's earlier study was to fixate on fat, specifically on how bad it was. The message became 'Get the fat out'. As a result, people were given advice such as 'Avoid oils' and 'Eat your salads dry if you can' and 'Use only fat-free salad dressings'. Moreover, because protein was a major source of fat in the diet, low fat often meant eating less red meat, chicken, fish and dairy and making up for it with lots of sugary and starchy refined carbohydrates.

The problem with the low-fat, high-carb recommendations was that they did not distinguish between good, high-fibre carbohydrates (such as whole fruits, vegetables and whole grains) and refined, low-fibre, high-sugar carbs (such as white bread and muffins). If the packaging said a food was 'low fat', it didn't matter if it had a high sugar or high starch content and virtually no nutrient value; it was considered to be okay.

The war on fat not only kept people away from bad saturated fat but led to the development of trans fats (which, in the form of partially hydrogenated oils, were invented to replace saturated fats like palm and coconut oils but turned out to be much worse). It also prevented them from getting the good, heart-healthy polyunsaturated omega-3 fatty acids found in cold-water fish and flaxseeds, for example, and the good, heart-healthy monounsaturated fats found in foods such as olive oil and nuts.

Through the 1980s and early 1990s, I watched my patients, the country, and frankly myself struggle with the so-called heart-healthy low-fat, high-carb diet. We tried our best to stick with it, but we were always hungry and rarely satisfied. What was even more distressing to me was that I saw problems in my patients' blood chemistries as we began to measure triglycerides and good HDL in addition to total cholesterol and LDL. I observed that some patients' triglycerides rose in response to the strict low-fat, high-carb diet they were following.

We now know that a high triglyceride level is often the body's response to excess sugar and starch in a person's diet. But back then, this wasn't well understood. To help my patients, I even tried the then-new, magic-bullet statin drugs lovastatin (Mevacor) and pravastatin (Lipostat), but the patients' triglyceride levels hardly budged. Furthermore, with the low-fat diet, their LDL cholesterol was also affected: it would go down a few points, which was good, but then it would return to baseline or go even higher. My experience with these patients was corroborated in the clinical trials I was reviewing at the time.

A Return to Sanity . . . and Satiety

Around the time I was seeing these problems with my patients, many advances in nutritional sciences were being reported, which greatly influenced my thinking. I began, for the first time in my medical career, to become optimistic and excited about the potential impact foods could have on health.

In 1995, based on the new nutritional information, I decided to try a good fats, good carbs, lean protein diet for myself and my patients. I was amazed by the results. For the first time, I saw their blood lipids, including their triglycerides, improve and their blood sugars normalize (as did my own). And, what's more, the fat in their bellies (and mine) seemed to melt away. Women excitedly reported their dress sizes going down, and men showed me tighter belt buckles to reveal their weight loss.

To find out how the good fats, good carbs approach stacked up against the old standard low-fat 'heart healthy' diet, my colleagues and I conducted a small clinical trial comparing our new approach with what was then called the Step II American Heart Association (AHA) Diet (their strictest low-fat diet at the time). In a group of 60 overweight participants, half went on our diet and the other half went on the Step II diet. After 12 weeks, five of the low-fat dieters had dropped out, but only one of the South Beach dieters had gone off the diet. Clearly, the low-fat diet was harder to swallow.

In the end, the South Beach dieters lost nearly twice as much weight as the low-fat dieters (a mean weight loss of 6 kg/13.6 lb compared to 3.4 kg/7.5 lb by the low-fat group). The South Beach dieters also showed a reduction in their really bad small, dense LDL cholesterol particles and an increase in LDL particle size, whereas the low-fat dieters did not. In addition, the South Beach Diet participants' triglycerides dramatically decreased, and their good-to-bad cholesterol ratio improved more than that of the low-fat group. But I've saved the best for last: the South Beach dieters lost more belly fat than the low-fat dieters, and as you know from reading Chapter 5, belly fat is an important risk factor for having a heart attack.

Does this study alone prove that the South Beach Diet is the best way to eat? The answer is 'No'. It is, in fact, the totality of evidence from hundreds of studies that proves that eating good fats, good carbs and lean protein is the best dietary approach to treating obesity, abnormal blood fats, and other heart-related problems.

The challenge in our society today is no longer to figure out what is good for us to eat or, for that matter, whether it is good for us to exercise. The challenge is to integrate healthy nutrition and regular exercise into our hectic everyday lives. While it would be ideal for us to return to family meals cooked from scratch after a hard day of physical labour, this is unlikely to happen. Instead, we have to incorporate good food and good amounts of exercise into the way we actually live. Helping you to accomplish this is my goal.

In spring 1999, after the presentation of some of our diet results at a national meeting of the American College of Cardiology in New Orleans, a Miami TV station asked us to put South Florida on the South Beach Diet. This was the moment when we moved from our clinical and research focus into the public sector as well. While all this happened quite serendipitously, it has given me the wonderful opportunity to help change the way people eat. Already there has been a substantial increase in awareness about good nutrition, and the beginnings of positive change are occurring in schools, restaurants and the food industry. I am delighted with this progress but know we have a long way to go.

How the South Beach Diet Helps Your Heart

How *does* the South Beach Diet help your heart? The answer is simple. Eating plenty of good unsaturated fats plays a role, as does enjoying lots of nutrient- and fibre-rich good carbs found in whole fruits, vegetables and whole grains. And, of course, weight loss – especially around our bellies – is a major factor for many people.

Good Fats and Your Heart

First, let's take a look at the good fats. Perhaps the most impressive heart disease prevention trial ever done was the Lyon Diet Heart Study, first reported in 1994. It tested the effect of a 'Mediterranean diet' on 605 patients who had already sustained a heart attack. Those on the Mediterranean diet were asked to eat more omega-3-rich oils (especially in the form of a rapeseed/canola oil spread), more olive oil and more fibre. The result: a dramatic 73 per cent decrease in heart attacks and other heart-related problems in those who ate this way – a decrease much greater than that seen in any previous or subsequent diet or single-medication trial. What's more, the benefits started very soon after the diet was initiated.

Of particular interest was that the decrease in heart attacks occurred without significant changes in cholesterol levels or in weight. It may be that the good fats make the lining of the heart's arteries healthier. They also make the blood less sticky and therefore less prone to developing large clots after vessel wall injury from plaque rupture. Since the Lyon study, there have been many other studies that have also demonstrated the lifesaving role good fats can play in heart disease. Studies also show that there are many noncardiac-related health benefits to eating good fats.

Good Carbs and Your Heart

As with the good fats, considerable research has established the role of good carbs in heart health. As I noted earlier, good carbs are vegetables, whole fruits and whole grains, which should be better represented in our diets not only in quantity but in quality and variety as well.

These foods are rich in phytochemicals, plant-based micronutrients that act in numerous ways – including as antioxidants – to improve our cardiovascular health and our health in general. Many studies show that antioxidants help protect us from free radicals, those aggressive, cell-damaging chemicals that can attack every component of the body, from the linings of our blood vessels to the retinas of our eyes.

We generate free radicals on a continual basis as a byproduct of the oxygen we use as fuel. We are also exposed to free radicals from external sources, such as ultraviolet rays from the sun, tobacco smoke, pollutants and other toxins. Free radicals are thought to play a major role in cardiovascular disease because they act in several ways to facilitate the formation of plaque. They also promote inflammation of the coronary arteries, which makes the lining of these vessels more susceptible to the rupture of soft plaque, which may result in a heart attack.

Plants need antioxidants to protect them from ultraviolet light and other threats to their survival. This is why fruits, vegetables and whole grains contain such a variety of phytochemicals. You may already know about some of them. Polyphenols, for example, are micronutrients found in green and white tea, red wine, dark chocolate, pomegranates and numerous other foods. Lycopene, a member of the carotenoid family, is found in such foods as tomatoes, pink and red grapefruit and papaya. Anthocyanins, which are purple to red in colour, are found in good amounts in blueberries, purple grapes, prunes, plums, aubergine (eggplant) and red wine. And lutein is found in spinach and other dark green leafy vegetables.

Weight Loss and Your Heart

Weight loss is one of the primary reasons the South Beach Diet can be expected to improve your cardiovascular health. Carrying around even a few pounds of excess weight can be taxing to your heart. For every pound you weigh, your body must develop millions of extra tiny blood vessels to feed it. If you were to take all of these blood vessels and place them in a straight line, it would add up to about 1 mile. So when you take off 5 pounds of fat, you are also losing 5 miles of blood vessels through which your heart would have to send blood (they are reabsorbed by the body). No wonder losing just a little weight can take stress off your heart and lower your blood pressure.

Weight loss will also improve your lipid numbers, particularly what I like to call your *lifestyle numbers*: your triglycerides and your good HDL. It will also decrease the dangerous fat stored in your belly. With

MAXIMIZING YOUR ANTIOXIDANTS

You may wonder which fruits and vegetables offer the most heart-protective antioxidant benefits. According to a rating of the antioxidant content in foods known as the ORAC scale (the acronym stands for Oxygen Radical Absorbance Capacity), compiled by the USDA, pomegranates have one of the highest antioxidant contents of all the fruits and vegetables that they measured.

While I usually recommend eating whole fruits as opposed to drinking fruit juice (juice doesn't usually contain much fibre and is high in sugar), I make an exception in the case of pomegranates. Studies have shown that 100 per cent pomegranate juice has unusual healing powers. In one study that used the thickness of the inner lining of the carotid artery wall to reflect atherosclerosis, there was literally a thinning of the wall in subjects who drank a glass of pomegranate juice daily. But as good as pomegranate juice is for you, I do suggest that you limit your intake to 60 to 120 ml (2 to 4 fl oz) a day and do not drink it until Phase 3 of the South Beach Diet (like all fruit juices, pomegranate juice does contain a fair amount of sugar). If you prefer to enjoy the seeds (which are allowed on Phase 2 of the diet), you can usually find the whole fruit in season (during the winter months) in your supermarket produce

a decrease in this fat, you reduce chronic inflammation, which is good for your heart, your brain and all your other organs as well.

The Role of Foods in Preventing Heart Disease

Within the past decade, we've learned a great deal about the roles that various foods – from apples to walnuts – play in preventing heart attack and stroke. Some foods are good at lowering bad LDL cholesterol and triglycerides, others help reduce blood pressure, and still others raise good HDL cholesterol.

Over the years, there has been some controversy over the benefits section. Sprinkle the seeds on a salad or over low-fat yogurt or cottage cheese or eat them directly from the fruit.

And which other fruits rate high on the antioxidant scale? The rule of thumb is that since antioxidants tend to concentrate in the skin, fruits with the highest ratio of skin to meat rate the highest. Therefore, all berries pack a strong antioxidant punch, with blueberries being the richest source. Plums, oranges, red grapes, cherries, kiwi fruit and pink and red grapefruit also rank high on the ORAC scale.

As far as vegetables are concerned, kale leads in the antioxidant ratings by far. Garlic, spinach, yellow squash, brussels sprouts, broccoli florets, avocados, red peppers (capsicums), aubergine (eggplant) and sweet potatoes are also high in antioxidants.

To date, more than 5000 different phytochemicals have been identified, and the list keeps growing. But when it comes to our knowledge of how these micronutrients actually protect our health, we've barely scratched the surface. At this time, these beneficial phytochemicals cannot be obtained from a vitamin pill. You need the whole food. Learning more about these substances will keep nutrition researchers busy for a long time.

of various foods for heart health. Take the good monounsaturated fat olive oil, for instance. While olive oil has been shown to help reduce the oxidation of LDL, making it less likely to invade your artery walls, whether it can actually lower LDL is subject to debate. That's because it is unclear whether it is the olive oil that is helping or simply the fact that people who eat olive oil also tend to avoid LDL-raising saturated fats and trans fats. To take another example, recent studies have found that the consumption of low-fat dairy products can help prevent high blood pressure. But there is no conclusive proof as to why. This has caused researchers to wonder whether it's the calcium content or some other unidentified components in the dairy products that are

OVERFED AND UNDERNOURISHED

You have probably heard the term *empty calories*. This refers to foods that contribute calories to your diet but have minimal nutrient value. These foods contain virtually no fibre, no vitamins, no minerals and none of the phytochemicals I discuss on pages 136–37. Pure starch-based foods, such as refined white flour, contribute empty calories, as do sugar, saturated fats and trans fats, which are devoid of nutrient value other than the energy gained from their calories. When we are consuming foods composed of empty calories, we are likely consuming fewer foods with the nutrients necessary for optimal health.

Often in medical science we can best appreciate the value of something when it has been taken away. When citrus fruits were absent from the diets of sailors in the 18th century, the sailors developed scurvy because of the lack of vitamin C. In many Western countries in the 20th century, we performed a similar unintentional experiment by taking the fibre and other healthy nutrients out of much of our food supply.

Although the problem of not getting enough good nutrients is fairly universal, we're seeing a particularly rapid rise in obesity and prediabetes in children, not to mention an increase in academic and behavioural problems, such as attention deficit disorder. This is not surprising when many of our children eat diets made up almost exclusively of starchy, sugary and trans fat-filled fast foods. These children, while seemingly overfed, are actually malnourished. And they are being set up for a host of health problems in the future.

But it's not just our children who are at risk. For adults, poor nutrition contributes not only to obesity, diabetes and heart disease, but to cancer, arthritis, Alzheimer's and many other chronic illnesses. If we continue to eat this way and allow our children to make bad food choices as well, we do so at our own peril.

providing the apparent benefits. I believe that future nutrition research will further elucidate these issues and solidify the roles of these and other foods in our cardiovascular and general health.

If you review the lists of 'Phase 1 Foods to Enjoy' on pages 152–55 and those that are added for Phase 2 of the South Beach Diet on pages 161–62, you will see many of the foods that have been found to have a positive effect on blood lipids. As you proceed through the diet's three phases, I urge you to eat more of these heart-protective foods on a daily basis. By making good food choices every day, you will feel satisfied and be less likely to eat the bad foods that increase your risk for heart disease.

Foods That Can Help Lower LDL

The good news – or the bad news, depending on what you're putting on your plate – is that bad LDL cholesterol is sensitive to diet (though less sensitive than triglycerides and HDL). Fortunately, the same foods that can help lower total LDL can also reduce the amount of small, dense LDL, which is the really bad cholesterol that burrows most easily into your artery walls and causes injury to the delicate linings. In addition, many of the foods that improve LDL also improve other blood lipids, including HDL and triglycerides.

Good LDL busters include:

Nuts and seeds. Sunflower seeds, pistachios, pumpkin seeds, sesame seeds, pine nuts, flaxseeds and almonds are particularly high in plant sterols, which can help reduce LDL. (For more on plant sterols, see pages 236–37.) Because it's easy to overdo it on nuts and seeds, limit your intake to about 30 g (1 oz) a day if you are also trying to lose weight.

Apples. Research shows that eating two apples a day can slow down the oxidation of LDL cholesterol and help prevent plaque buildup. The protective antioxidants are in the skin, so don't peel the apples.

Oat bran. An important source of water-soluble fibre, oats have long been recognized as a potential cholesterol-lowering dietary component. The soluble fibre in oat bran binds with bile acids in the intestine to block the absorption of cholesterol by the body. And according to a study conducted at the Jean Mayer USDA Human Nutrition Research Center on Aging in Boston, antioxidant compounds found in oat bran called *avenanthramides* can also prevent white blood cells from sticking to the artery walls, which is an important step in preventing plaque formation.

Tea. All varieties of antioxidant-rich tea (white, black, green, oolong) can help lower LDL, but oolong tea in particular has been found to increase LDL particle size. Oolong is the type of tea most commonly served in Chinese restaurants.

Grapefruit. Studies show that the phytochemicals called *liminoids* in pink and red grapefruit make them powerful LDL busters. Because grapefruit can interfere with the breakdown of certain medications, including statins and calcium channel blockers, check with your doctor before eating a lot of grapefruit or drinking the juice.

Monounsaturated oils. Olive oil and rapeseed (canola) oil, both good sources of monounsaturated fatty acids, can help lower LDL. But the effect on blood fats may be due, as I noted earlier, to the fact that people who eat monounsaturated fats in their diet often eat less saturated fats and trans fats. Monounsaturated fats are also anti-inflammatory and may help protect the lining of the coronary arteries (the *endothelium*) from inflammation, which is one of the ways that the delicate lining can be injured. As you may remember from Chapter 2, when the lining of the artery is injured, it allows LDL to enter, creating more plaque buildup.

Pulses. Kidney beans, soya beans, lentils, black beans and most other pulses are excellent sources of fibre and phytochemicals, which can help to lower LDL. In a study following more than 9600 men and women for 19 years, those who ate the most pulses had a 22 per cent lower risk of atherosclerosis and an 11 per cent lower risk of any kind of cardiovascular disease (such as stroke).

Foods That Can Help Raise HDL

HDL is the lipoprotein that shuttles excess cholesterol from plaque in the vessel walls back to the liver for excretion. It is easier to lower total cholesterol with diet than to raise HDL. In fact, the most effective way to raise HDL is to exercise and lose weight (especially belly fat).

Combining a diet high in good carbs and good fats with exercise and weight loss can have favourable and often dramatic effects on

HDL. Red wine and some other alcoholic beverages have also been found to increase HDL by themselves in patients who aren't overweight.

Good HDL boosters include:

Red wine. One or two 150 ml (5 fl oz) glasses of phytochemical-rich red wine daily (if you're not dieting or are on Phase 2 or 3 of the South Beach Diet) can raise HDL. Wine is a rich source of polyphenols, powerful antioxidants that protect the lining of the coronary arteries from free-radical injury.

But do stop at two glasses. More than two drinks daily may increase your risk of heart disease, as well as the risk of several types of cancer. Furthermore, alcohol is high in calories. If you need to lose weight, your intake of alcohol should be on an occasional basis.

Other alcoholic beverages. It is thought that beer, vodka and other alcoholic beverages may have the same favourable effects on HDL as wine. In fact, there are no good studies in real-world populations showing an advantage for wine over other alcoholic beverages. That said, I still prefer that my patients who want to have a drink choose wine because of its good polyphenol content. I also recommend that they have alcohol with meals to slow its absorption. Avoid mixed drinks and excessive intake.

Foods That Can Help Lower Triglycerides

High triglyceride levels are closely associated with prediabetes (metabolic syndrome), excess belly fat and low HDL. All are risk factors for heart attack and stroke. Eating a proper diet, losing weight if necessary and getting regular exercise can dramatically reduce triglyceride levels. In general, a high-fibre diet that's also rich in good omega-3 fatty acids can help lower triglyceride levels.

Good triglyceride busters include:

Oily fish. Of all the foods that can have a specific effect on lipids, omega-3-rich cold-water, oily fish are the most powerful when eaten by people with markedly elevated triglycerides. I have seen this many times in my own practice. Good choices include salmon, herring and sardines. Oily fish also contain natural blood thinners that can help prevent blood clots.

Nuts. Most nuts are sources of good fats, including omega-3s, but of all the nuts, walnuts are the richest in omega-3s. Walnuts are an excellent source of alpha-linolenic acid, a good plant-derived fat. A 2004 study in the *Journal of Nutrition* found that alpha-linolenic acid can decrease levels of C-reactive protein, a marker for inflammation. Keeping inflammation under control is especially important for people with prediabetes, which is associated with high triglycerides. Flaxseeds and flaxseed oil are also excellent sources of alpha-linolenic acid.

Whole grains. Eating plenty of whole grains is another way to protect against prediabetes and diabetes and the elevated triglycerides associated with these conditions. According to a recent study sponsored by the USDA, adults 60 years of age and older who ate three or more servings of whole grains daily (such as 100 per cent wholewheat bread, wholewheat pasta and brown rice) were significantly less likely to develop prediabetes than people who ate fewer servings.

Foods That Can Help Lower High Blood Pressure

First and foremost, if you are overweight and have high blood pressure, losing weight and getting regular exercise will help bring it down. If you've been eating a diet high in processed carbohydrates, exchanging those empty calories for high-fibre, nutrient-rich fruits, vegetables and whole grains; good fats; and lean protein – the foods I recommend on the South Beach Diet – will also help.

Recently, Johns Hopkins University conducted a study known as the Optimal Macronutrient Intake Trial to Prevent Heart Disease (also referred to as the OmniHeart trial). In the study, people with mildly high blood pressure replaced 10 per cent of their carbohydrate calories with lean protein calories that were specifically low in saturated fat. They did this by eating almonds, lean cuts of poultry and meat, black beans and egg substitute. Within 6 weeks, their blood pressure and cholesterol levels dropped significantly; and by the end of the study, the protein-enhanced diet had decreased the risk of cardiovascular disease by 21 per cent.

This is not to suggest that you should load up on meat and nothing else. In fact, in the OmniHeart trial, the participants ate *lean* protein, often from vegetable sources. (Other studies have shown that people who eat meat tend to have high blood pressure.) In fact, in study after study, it's the people who eat the most fruits and vegetables who have the lowest blood pressure. This is probably partly due to the fact that fruits and vegetables contain potassium, a mineral that has been shown to bring blood pressure down. But there are also scores of phyto-chemicals in fruits and vegetables that help relax blood vessel walls, allowing blood to flow more freely.

Often my patients ask me if cutting back on salt is a way to prevent high blood pressure. In reality, only about one-third to one-half of all people with high blood pressure are actually salt sensitive, which is defined as experiencing a greater than 10 per cent increase in blood pressure after eating a salty meal. If you know that you are salt sensi-tive, try to limit your sodium intake to 2300 mg daily, the equivalent of 1 teaspoon of salt.

Good blood pressure busters include:

Low-fat dairy. In a recent study of 5880 people, reported in the *American Journal of Clinical Nutrition*, participants who had the highest intake of low-fat milk and milk products had a 54 per cent reduced risk of developing high blood pressure. There appears to be a trend of positive research findings for low-fat dairy, including its ability to help promote weight loss and thus decrease the chance of diabetes.

Dark chocolate. Studies show that dark chocolate – not white chocolate or milk chocolate – increases the production of nitric oxide by the body, which dilates the large arteries, enhancing blood-flow and lowering blood pressure. Interestingly, the blood pressure-lowering effects of chocolate appear to be related to the amount of flavonoids present. Flavonoids are a type of polyphenol found natu-rally in the cocoa beans from which dark chocolate is made. Look for dark chocolate containing at least 70 per cent cocoa to reap the heart-health benefits. I tell my patients who are on Phase 2 or Phase 3 of the South Beach Diet that it can be healthy to enjoy chocolate once in a while. I certainly take my own advice – I'm an admitted chocoholic.

Whole grains, fruits, vegetables and pulses. People who eat plenty of plant foods have lower blood pressure, according to numerous studies. What do plant foods have in common? They're rich in heart-healthy phytochemicals that help keep arteries flexible and blood flowing optimally. But another common link is that most contain good amounts of fibre.

In a review published in the March 2005 issue of the *Journal of Hypertension*, researchers analysed 25 studies that looked at the effect of fibre on blood pressure. The results? Adding fibre-rich foods to the participants' diet caused a significant reduction in blood pressure among people with hypertension. Some good food sources of fibre are haricot beans, red kidney beans, black beans, wheat and oat bran, lentils, barley, sweet potatoes, pears, raspberries, blueberries, broccoli and wholemeal bread.

Red wine. A glass of red wine daily has been associated with lower blood pressure. Red wine contains resveratrol, a substance that helps to relax blood vessels and promote bloodflow. Larger amounts, however, can increase blood pressure in some people, so be moderate.

· · · · · · ·

By now I hope you're convinced that eating the right foods can make a difference in helping to prevent a heart attack or stroke. The more we study fruits, vegetables, whole grains, good fats and lean protein, the better they look. On the following pages, you will find the information you need to get started on the South Beach Diet – Step 1 to a heart-healthy way of life. You can also find menu plans, recipes and dietary advice in several of my other books. And, for even more support, visit our online centre at www.southbeachdiet.com/heart.

The South Beach Diet:
A Crash Course

The South Beach Diet is a blueprint for establishing the basic – and now widely agreed upon – nutritional principles for healthy eating in your own life. In my 10-plus years of experience with the diet, I have learned that the better you understand the rationale behind it, the better you will do. If you take the time to learn how the diet works and how it can help you maintain your health as you navigate through this busy world, you

THREE KEY PRINCIPLES OF
THE SOUTH BEACH DIET

1. Eat good fats. Choose good fats from olive oil, rapeseed (canola) oil, peanut oil, flaxseed oil, walnut oil, avocados, nuts and fish. Omega-3 (fish oil) supplements are also fine.

2. Eat good carbs. Good carbs include high-fibre, nutrient-dense fruits, vegetables, pulses and whole grains.

3. Eat lean protein. Eat eggs, low-fat dairy, nuts, seeds, pulses, white meat poultry, fish, shellfish and lean cuts of meat.

will have made great strides towards making healthy eating a way of life.

On the pages that follow, I review the principles of the diet and provide the information you need to get started right away. Once you understand its basic tenets, you can easily put together simple, healthy and delicious meals. Or, if you prefer, you can purchase prepared foods or eat out at restaurants. And even during Phase 1, the strictest part of the diet, there are always plenty of good food options that should keep you from feeling hungry or deprived. Best of all, once you have achieved your desired weight loss, there are no absolutely forbidden foods. You will know how to make the right food choices, and you can indulge in desserts and other special treats on occasion.

About the South Beach Diet Phases

The South Beach Diet is divided into three phases. Here's a quick summary of how each phase works, along with some sample meal plans and lists of foods to enjoy and foods to avoid in Phases 1 and 2.

PHASE 1

This is the shortest phase of the diet, lasting only 2 weeks. Phase 1 is for people who have significant cravings for refined starches and sugar or who have a substantial amount of weight to lose. It's also for those who are prediabetic or diabetic, which puts them at higher risk of having a heart attack or stroke. The purpose of this phase is to stabilize blood sugar levels and minimize those cravings. During this period, you will not be eating starches, including pasta, rice or bread of any type. You'll also eliminate sugar, even in fruits or fruit juices. Don't worry, you'll be able to eat these foods again when the 2 weeks are up. But trust me, you're not going to be hungry. During this time, you'll eat plenty of healthy foods, including lean protein (fish, chicken and lean cuts of beef), high-fibre vegetables, nuts, reduced-fat cheeses, eggs, low-fat dairy and good unsaturated fats such as olive oil and rapeseed (canola) oil. You'll eat three meals a day and at least two snacks. And you'll even be able to have some desserts, too! By the end of 2 short weeks, there will be a real difference in how you look and feel. You will have shed weight, but even more important, your blood chemistry will have improved and your cravings for the most part will be gone.

Many people lose weight fairly quickly on Phase 1. Quick weight loss can be a strong motivator, but it is important that this phase of the diet be limited in time. Those with predominant belly fat, pre-diabetes, high triglycerides and afternoon and evening cravings tend to lose weight the fastest. However, if people continue to lose weight at a rapid pace for weeks on end, they can develop a starvation reflex (one of the survival mechanisms I discussed in Chapter 5), which lowers their metabolism, slows weight loss and can lead to yo-yo dieting. For this reason, it is very important to move to Phase 2 after the first 2 weeks. Short-term weight loss is not the goal of the South Beach Diet. If you do not move on to the next phases, the diet will not become a lifestyle, and you are likely to regain lost weight.

On the next few pages, I have provided 2 days of sample meal plans for Phase 1, along with lists of foods to enjoy and foods to avoid during this phase. The wide variety of foods on the approved list allows you to mix and match foods to fit your own taste preferences.

For example, if you do not like broccoli, which I recommend for dinner on Day 1, substitute asparagus. Not a fan of salmon? Substitute fillet of sole for it on Day 2. Use these two meal plans as guidelines, then use the 'Phase 1 Foods to Enjoy' list to make your own menus for all 14 days of Phase 1.

Keep in mind that the South Beach Diet doesn't require you to measure what you eat in grams, calories or anything else. Weighing, measuring and counting are certainly not conducive to a pleasant lifestyle, and it is an approach you're unlikely to sustain. It is also unnecessary. Generally, if you are making the right food choices, portion control takes care of itself. Your meals should be of normal size – enough to satisfy your hunger. And while you should never leave a meal hungry, that doesn't mean that you must clean your plate. Try to eat slowly so that your brain has time to detect your normal rise in blood sugar. This is difficult to do if you have allowed cravings to occur. It becomes much easier once you have completed Phase 1 and cravings have largely disappeared.

But while I don't recommend weighing and measuring, I do recommend that you eat a minimum of 200 g (7 oz) of vegetables with lunch and dinner so you get the maximum heart-protective antioxidant and fibre benefits. Remember to drink water and keep yourself hydrated throughout the day.

(See Sample Meal Plans and food lists on the following pages.)

DAY 1

BREAKFAST

180 ml (6 fl oz) vegetable juice cocktail

Scrambled eggs with spinach and mushrooms

Turkey bacon or lean back bacon

Coffee or tea with skimmed milk and sugar substitute

MIDMORNING SNACK

Fat-free natural yogurt with almond extract, sugar substitute and toasted almonds

LUNCH

Warm sliced sirloin steak with spring greens and no-sugar-added balsamic dressing

Black bean, avocado and tomato salad

MIDAFTERNOON SNACK

Hummus with vegetable crudité

DINNER

Spicy grilled chicken and red onion kebabs

Sautéed broccoli with olives

Cucumber, radish and feta salad with dill vinaigrette

DESSERT

No-sugar-added ice-lolly with a glass of skimmed milk

DAY 2

BREAKFAST

180 ml (6 fl oz) tomato juice

Spanish omelette

Lean back bacon

Coffee or tea with skimmed milk and sugar substitute

MIDMORNING SNACK

115 g (4 oz) naturally fat-free cottage cheese with chopped spring onions

LUNCH

Lentil soup

Curried chicken salad with water chestnuts

Red leaf lettuce salad with Dijon vinaigrette

MIDAFTERNOON SNACK

15 almonds and a glass of skimmed milk

DINNER

Grilled salmon steak with lemon and capers

Steamed asparagus with shaved Parmesan

Warm cannellini or haricot beans with rosemary

DESSERT

Reduced-fat ricotta whisked with a dash of vanilla, sugar substitute and a sprinkling of almonds

BEEF

Lean* cuts, such as:

    Fillet

    Sirloin

    Topside

Ground beef:

    Extra lean

    Lean

    Sirloin

Pastrami, lean

Rump (trimmed of fat)

T-bone

*Lean meat has 10 g or less of total fat and 4.5 g or less of saturated fat per 100 g portion.

POULTRY (skinless)

Turkey bacon

Turkey or chicken breast

Guinea fowl

Poussin

SEAFOOD

All types of fish and shellfish (limit those high in mercury, such as swordfish, shark and marlin)

Salmon roe

Sashimi

PORK

Boiled ham

Lean back bacon

Loin (trimmed of fat)

Tenderloin/fillet

VEAL

Chops, cutlets (trimmed of fat)

Escalopes

LAMB (remove all visible fat)

Leg or leg steaks

Loin chops

COLD MEATS
(fat-free or low-fat only)

Boiled ham

Turkey breast

Roast beef (topside)

Smoked ham

SOYA-BASED MEAT SUBSTITUTES

Unless otherwise stated, look for products that have 6 g or less of fat per 60–90 g (2–3 oz) serving.

Bacon

Burger

Chicken, unbreaded

Hot dogs

Sausages

Tempeh – 40 g (1¾ oz) suggested serving size

Tofu (all varieties) 125 g (4½ oz) suggested serving size

CHEESE (fat-free or reduced-fat)

For hard cheese, look for varieties that have 6 g or less of fat per 30 g (1 oz) serving.

Cheddar

Cottage cheese, virtually or fat-free

Feta

Mozzarella

Parmesan

Ricotta

String cheese

Swiss

EGGS

The use of whole eggs is not limited unless otherwise directed by your doctor. Egg whites and egg substitutes are okay.

DAIRY

480 ml (16 fl oz) allowed daily, including natural fat-free or low-fat yogurt.

Milk, skimmed

Soya milk, low-fat plain, vanilla, or sucralose-containing (4 g or less of fat per 230 g/8 oz serving). Be sure that the product does not contain high-fructose corn syrup.

Yogurt, low-fat or fat-free natural

PULSES

Start with a 60–90 g (2–3 oz) serving size.

Aduki beans

Black beans

Black-eyed peas

Broad beans

Butter beans

Cannellini beans

Chickpeas

Edamame (soya beans)

Flageolet beans

Haricot beans

Kidney beans

Lentils

Mung beans

Split peas

VEGETABLES

May use fresh, frozen or canned without added sugar. Eat a minimum of 200 g (7 oz) with lunch and dinner.

Artichokes

Asparagus

Aubergine (eggplant)

Avocados

Broccoli

Brussels sprouts

Cabbage

Capers

Cauliflower

Celery

Cucumbers

Endive

Fennel

Garlic

Green beans

Greens (all varieties)

Hearts of palm

Kale

Leeks

Lettuce (all varieties)

Mangetout

Mushrooms (all varieties)

Okra

Onions

Pak choi (bok choy)

Parsley

Peppers (all varieties)

Pickles (dill or artificially sweetened)

Radicchio

Radishes

Rhubarb

Rocket

Sauerkraut

Sea vegetables

Spinach

Spring onions

Sprouts, alfalfa

Squash

Sugar snap peas

Swiss chard

Tomatoes

Tomato juice

Vegetable juice cocktail

Water chestnuts

Watercress

NUTS AND SEEDS

*Limit to one serving per day as
specified. Unsalted
recommended.*

Almonds – 15

Brazil nuts – 4

Cashews – 15

Flaxseed – 3 Tbs (30 g/1 oz)

Hazelnuts – 25

Macadamias – 8

Peanut butter, natural and other
nut butters – 2 Tbs

Peanuts – 20 small (dry roasted
or boiled)

Pecans – 15

Pine nuts – 30 g (1 oz)

Pistachios – 30

Pumpkin seeds – 3 Tbs (30 g/1 oz)

Sesame seeds – 3 Tbs (30 g/
1 oz)

Soya nuts – 3 Tbs (30 g/1 oz)

Sunflower seeds – 3 Tbs (30 g/
1 oz)

Walnuts – 15

FATS AND OILS

*Up to 2 tablespoons of the
following fats or oils are allowed
daily. Monounsaturated oils are
particularly recommended.*

Monounsaturated Oils

Olive oil (particularly extra-virgin)

Rapeseed (canola) oil

Polyunsaturated Oils or a
Blend of Monounsaturated
and Polyunsaturated

Corn

Flaxseed

Grapeseed

Peanut

Safflower

Sesame

Soya bean

Sunflower

Other Fat Choices

Avocado – ⅓ whole = 1 Tbs oil

Guacamole – 115 g (4 oz) = 1
Tbs oil

Margarine – those that do not
contain trans fatty acids

Mayonnaise, regular – 1 Tbs

Mayonnaise, low-fat – 2 Tbs
(avoid varieties made with high-
fructose corn syrup)

Olives (green or ripe) – 15 = ½
Tbs oil

Salad dressing – 2 Tbs. Use
those that contain 3 g of sugar
or less per 2 Tbs. Best choices
contain rapeseed (canola) or
olive oil. Dressings labelled
'low-carb' may only be used if
they meet these guidelines.

Trans fat-free spreads

SEASONINGS AND CONDIMENTS

All spices that contain no added sugar

Espresso powder

Extracts (almond, vanilla or others)

Horseradish sauce

Lemon juice

Lime juice

Pepper (black, cayenne, chilli, white)

Salsa (check label for added sugar)

Stock

Use the following toppings and sauces sparingly; check label for added sugar or monosodium glutamate (MSG):

Cream cheese, fat-free or light – 2 Tbs

Hot sauce

'Low-carb' condiments may only be used if they are trans-fat free and contain no added sugar.

Miso – ½ Tbs

Shoyu – ½ Tbs

Soured cream, light or reduced-fat – 2 Tbs

Soy sauce – ½ Tbs

Tamari – 1 Tbs

Worcestershire sauce – 1 Tbs

Whipped topping, light – 2 Tbs

SWEET TREATS

Limit to 75–100 calories/315–420 kilojoules per day.

Chewing gum, sugar-free

Cocoa powder, unsweetened

Ice-lollies, sugar-free

Jams, sugar-free

Jelly, sugar-free

Sweets, hard, sugar-free

Some sugar-free products may be made with sugar alcohols (isomalt, lactitol, mannitol, sorbitol or xylitol) and are permitted on the South Beach Diet.

SUGAR SUBSTITUTES

Acesulfame K

Fructose (count as Sweet Treats, 75–100 calorie/315–420 kilojoule limit)

Aspartame (NutraSweet, Equal)

Saccharin (Sweet'N Low)

Sucralose (Splenda)

Some sugar substitutes may be made with sugar alcohols (isomalt, lactitol, mannitol, sorbitol or xylitol) and are permitted on the South Beach Diet.

BEVERAGES

Decaffeinated coffee and tea

Diet, decaffeinated, sugar-free drinks

Herbal teas (peppermint, chamomile, etc.)

Milk, skimmed

Soya milk, low-fat plain, vanilla or sucralose-containing (4 g or less of fat per 240 ml/8 fl oz serving). Be sure that the product does not contain high-fructose corn syrup.

Sugar-free powdered drink mixes

Vegetable juice

Note: Caffeinated coffee, regular tea and diet drinks with caffeine added are allowed, but limited to one or two servings per day.

PHASE 1 FOODS TO AVOID

BEEF
Brisket

Liver

Prime rib

Rib steak

POULTRY
Chicken, wings and legs

Duck

Goose

Poultry products, processed

Turkey, dark meat (including wings and thighs)

PORK
Honey-baked ham

Streaky bacon

VEAL
Breast

DAIRY
Ice cream

Milk, Semi-skimmed or whole

Soya milk, whole

Yogurt, regular and frozen

CHEESE
Full-fat

FRUITS
Avoid all fruits and fruit juices on Phase 1

VEGETABLES
Beetroot

Carrots

Parsnips

Peas, green

Potatoes, sweet

Potatoes, white

Pumpkin

Sweetcorn

Turnips (root)

Yams

STARCHES
Avoid all starchy food on Phase 1, including:

Bread, all types

Cereal

Croutons, all types

Matzo

Oats

Pasta, all types

Pastries and baked goods, all types

Rice, all types

MISCELLANEOUS
Cocktail sauce

Ketchup

BEVERAGES
No alcohol of any kind, including beer and wine

PHASE 2

Those people who have 4.5 kg (10 lb) or less to lose, who don't have problems with cravings, who don't have excess belly fat, or who simply want to improve their health can start the diet with Phase 2.

If you're moving into Phase 2 from Phase 1, you'll be reintroducing foods that were off-limits on Phase 1, including healthy carbs such as wholemeal bread, brown rice, whole-wheat pasta, whole fruits and some root vegetables (such as sweet potatoes). You will also be able to have a glass or two of red or white wine with meals and even the occasional piece of dark chocolate, if you like.

The key to continuing your weight loss on Phase 2 is to reintroduce these foods gradually, so you can monitor your hunger and possible cravings. For example, you can begin Phase 2 by having one whole-grain food and one fruit each day for the first few days in addition to your lean protein, vegetables and low-fat dairy. If you continue to lose weight, you can gradually add more fruits, whole grains and other foods from the 'Foods to Reintroduce in Phase 2' list on pages 161–62. You will continue Phase 2 until you reach a weight that's healthy for you.

Remember that this is a slower weight-loss phase than Phase 1: losing 0.5–1 kg (1–2 lb) per week on Phase 2 is fine. Gradual weight loss over a long period of time leads to permanent weight loss, so do not get impatient. The best indicator that the diet is working is the absence of cravings, not faster weight loss. If the cravings return, you should become more strict. And be sure to exercise! It will improve your results and is a critical component of the South Beach Diet lifestyle.

· · · · · · ·

On the next few pages, I have provided two days of Sample Meal Plans for Phase 2 followed by a list of heart-healthy foods you can now add to those you already enjoyed on Phase 1. There is also a list of a few foods to continue to avoid on Phase 2. The Day 1 Meal Plan gives you an idea of what you might eat on the first few days or weeks of Phase 2; the Day 2 Meal Plan illustrates a typical day further into

Phase 2, when you've added more fruit and other carbohydrates, as I described earlier. Both days' meals are designed to be high in heart-healthy fats, fibre and heart-protective phytochemicals.

A note about whole grains: In Phase 2, you will be introducing whole grains into your diet, but I want you to purchase the right ones. When you buy wholemeal breads and other products, be sure the label says '100 per cent whole wheat', 'wholemeal' or 'whole grain', not 'enriched' or 'fortified' grain or simply '100 per cent wheat' or 'multigrain'. The process of refining white flour depletes it of much of its fibre and nutrients. Food manufacturers often add back some of these nutrients and label the product 'enriched' or 'fortified'. Enriched and/or fortified products are no substitute for the real thing. Stick to 100 per cent whole-wheat or whole-grain products.

(See Sample Meal Plans and food lists on the following pages.)

DAY 1

BREAKFAST

180 ml (6 fl oz) vegetable juice cocktail

Rolled oats with cinnamon

Low-fat or fat-free natural or artificially sweetened yogurt

Coffee or tea with skimmed milk and sugar substitute

MIDMORNING SNACK

1 boiled egg with a slice of lean ham

LUNCH

Gazpacho

Seared tuna with chickpeas on a bed of greens

MIDAFTERNOON SNACK

1 slice mozzarella light

DINNER

Pan-grilled sirloin steak with sautéed mushrooms and onions

Steamed green beans with garlic and lemon

Hearts of romaine with toasted pistachios and pomegranate seeds (in season)

Extra-virgin olive oil and vinegar

DESSERT

Dark chocolate-dipped strawberries

DAY 2

BREAKFAST

½ pink or red grapefruit

1 egg, poached or any style

1 slice 100% wholemeal toast with virtually fat-free cottage cheese, cinnamon and a sprinkling of sugar substitute

Coffee or tea with skimmed milk and sugar substitute

MIDMORNING SNACK

Whole-wheat crackers with 1 wedge spreadable reduced-fat cheese

LUNCH

Grilled prawn Caesar salad

Sliced pear with crumbled gorgonzola

MIDAFTERNOON SNACK

15 walnuts and a glass of skimmed milk

DINNER

Garlic-rubbed grilled lamb chop

Baked sweet potato

Sautéed kale with shallots

Tomato salad with fresh basil, extra-virgin olive oil and vinegar

DESSERT

Baked apple with fat-free natural yogurt

You can enjoy all the foods on Phase 1, as well as those listed on this and the following page:

BEEF

All hot dogs and soya sausages can be enjoyed occasionally (once a week) if they are at least 97% fat free (3–6 g of fat per serving).

FRUIT

Start with one serving daily, gradually increasing to up to three servings daily.

Apple – 1 small or 5 dried rings

Apricots – 4 fresh or 7 dried

Banana – 1 medium (115 g/ 4 oz)

Berries, all – 90 g (3 oz)

Cantaloupe – ¼ melon

Cherries – 12

Grapefruit – ½

Grapes – 15

Kiwi fruit – 1

Mango – ½ medium (115 g/4 oz)

Orange – 1 medium

Papaya – 1 small (115 g/4 oz)

Peach – 1 medium

Pear – 1 medium

Plums – 2

Prunes – 4

Tangerines – 2

VEGETABLES

Carrots – 75 g (2½ oz)

Peas, green – 75 g (2½ oz)

DAIRY

480–720 ml (16–26 fl oz) allowed daily, including yogurt.

Yogurt – 115 g (4 oz) per day (artificially sweetened low-fat or fat-free flavoured yogurt; avoid varieties that contain high-fructose corn syrup).

WHOLE GRAINS AND STARCHY VEGETABLES

Start with one serving daily, gradually increasing to up to three or four servings daily. Unless otherwise stated, choose whole-grain products that have 3 g or more of fibre per serving.

Bagels, whole grain – ½ small (30 g/1 oz)

Barley – 75 g (2½ oz) cooked

Bread – 1 slice (30 g/1 oz)

> homemade breads made with whole grains (buckwheat, whole wheat, spelt, whole oats, bran, rye)
>
> multigrain
>
> oat and bran
>
> rye
>
> sprouted grain
>
> wholemeal

Buckwheat – 75 g (2½ oz) cooked

Cereal, hot (choose whole-grain and slow-cooking varieties, not instant)

Cereal, cold (choose low-sugar with 5 g or more of fibre per serving)

Couscous or bulgar wheat –
75 g (2½ oz) cooked

Crackers, whole grain (3 g or
more of fibre per 30 g and no
trans fats)

English muffin, whole grain –
½ muffin. Most contain 2.5 g of
fibre per half a muffin – varieties
with 3 g of fibre are the best
choice

Green peas – 75 g (2½ oz)
(considered a starchy
vegetable, count as a starch/
grain serving)

Muffin, bran – 1 small, homemade
sugar-free, no raisins

Pasta

> whole wheat – 75 g (2½
> oz) cooked (3 g or more of
> fibre per 75 g/2½ oz)

> soya – 90 g (3 oz) cooked
> (3 g or more of fibre per
> 90 g/3 oz)

Pitta – ½ pitta (30 g/1 oz). Most
contain 2.5 g of fibre per half
pitta – varieties with 3 g of fibre
are the best choice

> stone-ground

> whole wheat

Popcorn – 30 g (1 oz) popped

> air popped

> microwave, plain, no trans fats

> stove-top, cooked with
> rapeseed (canola) oil

Potato, sweet, 1 small (considered
a starchy vegetable, count as a
starch/grain serving)

Pumpkin – 90 g (3 oz)
(considered a starchy
vegetable, count as a starch/
grain serving)

Quinoa – 75 g (2½ oz) cooked

Rice – 75 g (2½ oz) cooked

> basmati

> brown, regular, or
> parboiled

> wild

Rice noodles – 90 g (3 oz)
cooked

Soba noodles – 90 g (3 oz)
cooked

Squash, winter – 100 g (3½ oz)
(considered a starchy
vegetable, count as a starch/
grain serving)

Tortilla, 100% whole grain –
1 small (3 g or more of fibre
per 30 g, no trans fats)

Yam – 1 small (considered a
starchy vegetable, count as a
starch/grain serving)

OCCASIONAL TREATS

Chocolate (limited)

> plain, dark

Sugar-free jelly (one serving per
day permitted)

BEVERAGES

Wine, red or white (1–2 glasses
permitted daily with or after meals)

PHASE 2 FOODS TO AVOID OR EAT RARELY

STARCHES

Bagel, refined wheat flour

Biscuits

Bread

    refined wheat flour

    white

Cornflakes

Matzo (except whole-wheat varieties, which are allowed)

Pasta, white flour

Potatoes

    white

    instant

Rice cakes

Rice

    white

    jasmine

    sticky

Rolls, white dinner

FRUIT

Canned fruit, in heavy syrup

Fruit juice

Pineapple

Raisins

Watermelon

VEGETABLES

Beetroot

Potatoes, white

Sweetcorn

MISCELLANEOUS

Honey

Ice cream

Jam

PHASE 3

Phase 3 begins once you reach your healthy weight. Obviously, with your newfound confidence about making good food choices, you'll continue to eat the right carbs, the right fats, lean sources of protein, low-fat dairy and plenty of fibre. At this point, you'll fully understand what you can eat while still maintaining your health and your weight. Since your South Beach Diet lifestyle will be second nature and you'll be able to monitor your body's response to particular foods with ease, you'll find yourself enjoying foods of all types – including the occasional empty-calorie indulgence – whether you're cooking at home for yourself and your family, ordering in, or dining out.

What if you start to regain a lot of weight on Phase 3? If this is associated with cravings or your doctor tells you that your cholesterol and triglycerides are on the rise, you may want to return to Phase 1 for several days until your cravings resolve. This will help. If your weight gain is minimal and you don't have cravings, simply return to a Phase 2 eating plan that worked for you before. The beauty of the South Beach Diet is that it's flexible enough to accommodate the normal changes of daily life.

Melanie's Story

'My blood pressure was 190/120. When my doctor saw that, he said, "I'm really afraid for you right now."'

I first heard about the South Beach Diet at the medical clinic where I work. I'm a receptionist for a general practitioner. He had a number of his patients on the diet and they were doing really well. I was 36 kg (80 lb) overweight and was beginning to think I should do something about it. At the time, I had high cholesterol and acid reflux. What really got me motivated was the day I went to my own doctor and found out that my blood pressure was 190/120. When my doctor saw that, he said, 'I'm really afraid for you right now. I don't want you to leave here without blood pressure medication.' He didn't tell me to lose weight, but I knew that I had to.

When I started the diet, I was taking two different hypertension drugs, a statin and an antireflux medication. I was also taking antidepressants because I was under a lot of stress. My husband was out of work and my mother had just died. She'd had her first heart attack when she was only 53, followed by quadruple bypass surgery. She was 56 when she died of a massive heart attack. She was obese – I'd say 45 kg (100 lb) overweight. She was also diabetic. And she smoked. Every woman in my family is obese and diabetic except for one cousin who works on a farm.

But for years and years, I didn't eat fat. No oil or anything. Completely fat-free dressings. I wasn't getting the good fats, and I was really into sugar. I would eat a whole box of fat-free biscuits. I figured, there's no fat in it, so it's okay. I kept eating a low-fat diet even when I was gaining weight instead of losing it. It's the only diet that people recommended.

I started the South Beach Diet in January of 2005. I found it very easy. I didn't have any trouble on Phase 1 until 3 days before the end. Then I really wanted some rice. Really bad. But I didn't want sugar anymore and that was amazing. People were already commenting on my weight loss – I had lost 5 kg (11 lb) – because they could see it in my face.

Phase 2 was easier, and it wasn't. It was easier because there was a lot more I could eat. But it was hard to give up the strictness of Phase 1, because I had lost so much weight. I was afraid that if I started eating more carbohydrates, I wouldn't keep losing. But I did. My weight loss slowed down, but it never stopped.

Just 8 months into the diet, I had lost 18 kg (40 lb), and I no longer needed any medications. I stopped taking the blood pressure medication because my blood pressure was getting too low. I never thought I'd see the end of acid reflux, but it was completely gone. I didn't know if it was just because my stomach was smaller or because I was eating healthier food. Right now, I'm only taking a fish oil supplement and I'm really happy. ■

STEP
2

THE SOUTH BEACH
HEART WORKOUT

The second step of the South Beach Heart Programme is about *literally* taking steps to protect your heart. It's about getting out of your chair or off your sofa and taking a walk every day. It's about devoting some time each day to stretching and strengthening your muscles. It's about living pain free and injury free. It's about staying trim and standing straight and tall. It's about making exercise a regular part of your life in order to extend your life. And, finally, it's about exercising your body the way it was designed to be exercised.

The South Beach Heart Workout is my exercise prescription for a healthy heart and a healthy body. The workout consists of an easy, yet comprehensive two-part functional fitness regime that can be done anytime, anywhere, and can easily be worked into your busy schedule. It doesn't require any special equipment, and it emphasizes the components of total fitness.

The first part of the workout involves walking, an aerobic form of exercise that nearly everyone can do. Not only is walking good for every muscle in your body, when it is done at the right pace, it gets your heart pumping and your blood flowing. That's why aerobics is sometimes referred to as *cardio conditioning*. A good aerobic workout will strengthen your heart and make it much easier for it to perform its normal workload.

The second part of the workout emphasizes strengthening the *core* muscles of the trunk of your body (your abdomen, lower back, pelvis and hips), which is essential for properly strengthening your peripheral muscles. The core muscles support all your other muscles and help you maintain good posture and balance. More important, your core muscles help keep you stable. You may wonder why a cardiologist would be concerned about strengthening muscles other than the heart muscle. The answer is simple – you can't keep your heart strong and your body healthy if your other muscles are weak.

You may not think of yourself as a risk taker, but being sedentary is as much of a risk factor for heart disease as smoking or having high blood pressure. And yet, despite the risk, physical inactivity has become a way of life for many of us. Recent statistics show that 70 per cent of the adult population is sufficiently inactive to be classed as sedentary. It's hardly a coincidence that 1 in 5 of UK adults are obese.

Not surprisingly, by the time all these couch potatoes reach middle age, their core muscles are so out of shape that they are likely to suffer from a litany of ailments rooted in this weakness. If you sat in on some of my patient interviews every day, you would hear complaints like these: 'My back hurts all the time!' 'My knee is so sore I can't walk up the steps.' 'My shoulder is so stiff.' I take these complaints very seriously. When someone is in pain, that person is less likely to walk or do any exercise, aerobic or otherwise. This, in turn, creates a vicious cycle: the less activity you do, the weaker your muscles become and the more prone you are to injury. The weaker your muscles become, the more likely you are to hurt, and then you cut back on your activities even further. This lack of activity means you're not burning many calories during the day, which will ultimately result in weight gain, obesity, diabetes and potentially a heart attack or stroke.

So that's why a cardiologist is so interested in core training! And that's why you should be, too.

Exercise for the Real World

The South Beach Heart Workout emphasizes functional fitness. That's because I strongly believe that one of the main goals of an exercise programme should be to improve your ability to function in the real world. The core exercises and walking plan I recommend can be done at home and throughout the day and will make it easier for you to perform your normal daily activities, whether that involves lifting a child, lugging shopping bags from your car to your house, or running to catch a train. In addition, this fitness plan will help keep you injury free, which is the key to staying active and living a longer, happier and heart-healthy life.

It's well known that conventional weight training, which is how many people exercise, tends to isolate muscle groups and focus more on strengthening the arms and legs than on improving the core muscles. In fact, most methods of weight training do not require you to use several muscle groups in one fluid movement. Many gym-goers who can bench press a heavy weight can't hoist an 18-kg (40-lb) bag of dog food from the shopping trolley to the car without experiencing back pain. They have been neglecting their back and stomach muscles. *Integration* is the underlying principle of functional exercise. You need to strengthen and stretch *all* of your muscles and train them to work together so you stay out of pain.

We Weren't Always Sedentary

Not so long ago, people didn't have to go to the gym or perform special exercises to stay fit. The demands of daily living accomplished this goal. A farmer who pitched hay used his arms, legs, shoulders, buttocks and torso in one continuous movement. A woman scrubbing clothes on a washboard and hanging them to dry on a clothesline was toning and stretching her entire upper body. Chopping wood, tilling the garden and harvesting crops were full-body activities. During all of these movements, while the arms were moving, the core muscles were working hard to maintain good posture. You simply could not pitch hay for very long with a rounded rather than a straight back, so good posture was a natural consequence of performing such functional chores. Today, with our sedentary lifestyles, most people have to make a special effort to develop their major muscle groups and keep them supple and flexible.

I had firsthand experience with the need to strengthen my core muscles when our first son was nearly a year old. He had a little trouble falling asleep, and my wife, Sari, and I found that carrying him in our arms on long evening walks helped. It became an evening ritual that we dubbed 'The Evan Shuffle'. Even though I was lifting weights at the time, I quickly found that carrying my son for half an hour every night really put a strain on my lower back. I remember straightening up and trying to improve my posture as I walked because it took some of the stress off my back. In fact, I was forced into having good posture during this period of baby-induced 'functional training', because weight training using machines hadn't made my stomach and back muscles as strong as I thought.

After a few weeks of walking with Evan and concentrating on my posture, I discovered that my back didn't ache anymore and that I was noticeably stronger. At about that time, we moved to a new house, and I had to load and move a lot of heavy boxes. I was surprised to see how easily I could lift them without straining, and I wasn't even winded. Conditioning my core muscles and building my endurance by carrying my son every night had made a big difference in other aspects of my life as well. And thankfully, Evan finally learned to sleep through the night.

A Little Goes a Long Way

I know that many of you are thinking, 'Sure I'd like to exercise, but I don't have the time.' As you will learn, it doesn't require that much time to stay reasonably fit while significantly reducing your risk of heart disease. According to the Framingham Heart Study, which I discussed in Chapter 3, and many other heart studies as well, walking briskly for 30 minutes a day – even for people who take up this form of exercise later in life – can increase life expectancy by years. More important, those bonus years have been shown to be virtually free of heart disease.

Even simply staying active throughout the day can be lifesaving. The husband of one of my patients is a good example. Jerold is 84 years old. He's tall, lean and has a ruddy complexion. His wife, Maryanne, is 78. She is overweight, has diabetes and had two heart attacks before she became my patient. Although she's 6 years younger than Jerold, she looks and acts much older.

I asked Jerold about his own health one day when he came into the office with Maryanne. He told me that his cholesterol and blood pressure were low and that he had never had any weight or heart problems. I asked him what his secret was, and he said he just keeps busy. 'I take the dog for a walk in the morning. I come home and do the housework and the yard work. All day I take care of Maryanne. I walk the dog again after dinner. I figure that if I keep moving, they can't bury me.'

There's much truth to Jerold's remark, especially when it comes to weight creep, the slow but insidious weight gain people often experience as they age. Recent studies suggest that staying active may be the key to keeping off extra weight as we get older – in fact, it may be as important, if not more important, than going on a diet. Just getting up and moving burns calories. And you don't have to run marathons to get the benefit: even activities such as gardening or doing housework count. Keep in mind that if you burn just a few hundred extra calories a day, over the course of a year, this could add up to a loss of at least several pounds. And it will also help you keep off weight that you've already lost. Even more important, since obesity is a major risk factor for heart disease, staying trim helps to keep your heart healthy.

Everything to Lose

Why is inactivity such a threat to your heart health? Here's the nutshell explanation. As you age, you lose a little bone and muscle with each passing year. This is due to decreasing levels of the sex hormones oestrogen and testosterone. Your body composition shifts, and extra calories that aren't being used to maintain bone and muscle are stored as fat, often in the belly (in fact, in just 6 months of inactivity, belly fat can increase by as much as 9 per cent!). The more fat in your belly, the more insulin it takes to withdraw sugar from your bloodstream and store it as energy. As I discussed in Chapter 5, when your blood levels of sugar creep upwards, more fat begins to hang around in your blood in the form of triglycerides. You also have more of the dangerous small, dense LDL cholesterol that invades your arteries. Your entire system becomes more inflamed, and you become more vulnerable to blood clot formation. Meanwhile, your blood pressure has been climbing as well. First you enter the prehypertension zone and, before you know it, you may 'graduate' to full-blown hypertension. And all you did was sit there.

The Core Busters

Over time, civilization has created what I like to call 'core busters' because they rob our core muscles of the activities they were meant to experience. In fact, the first core buster was probably the chair.

If you have seen pictures of contemporary men and women from primitive cultures, you might notice that they easily squat or sit on the ground with a straight back. That's because their core muscles haven't been busted yet. Today, toddlers sitting on the floor playing with toys do the same thing. They sit up with a straight back because their muscles are strong. It's only when these children begin sitting on chairs that the weakening of their core muscles begins.

While industrialization in the late 1800s certainly began a decline in physical activity, the weakening of our core has been greatly accelerated in the last half century with the advent of so many automated appliances, including the TV. But today it's not the TV that's the ultimate core buster. It's the personal computer. Thanks to the computer revolution, we can tap away at the keyboard to take care of most of our needs and never get up from our chair. Mind you, I love the computer, but think about it: today we can order pizza, shop, download music, stay in touch with family and friends, find a mate, get parenting advice, plan our holidays, pay our bills, save for retirement, order medications, even sign up for a burial plot without ever standing up. To add insult to injury, when we sit in front of the computer for long hours doing all this, we're leaning forwards, hunched over, weakening our back and our abdominal muscles.

When we move too little, our bodies cease to function as nature intended. To get back in shape and reduce the risk of cardiovascular disease, we have to make a conscious effort to exercise. I certainly try to practise what I preach. Like many people, my life is very busy and I have little free time. If I'm going to exercise, I have to make time to do it (usually early in the morning). But when I do exercise regularly, I feel great and look better for it.

As with diet, the challenge with exercise is sticking with it. You don't need a gym to make walking and other exercise a daily habit. In fact, sometimes the pressure of travelling to a gym can actually make people feel less like exercising. (I've often been impressed by the business strategy gyms employ when they offer great long-term deals for signing up. They know that most people will not use their membership beyond the short-term.) Don't get me wrong. I believe that the proliferation of gyms is a positive sign that we are becoming more exercise conscious. So, if you can make trips to the gym part of your lifestyle, great. Trainers at gyms can be very helpful in inspiring you and making sure you are exercising safely and correctly. But if trips to the gym don't fit into your lifestyle, you can still be successful. US studies show that for preventing weight gain and heart disease, inhabitants of walking cities such as New York and San Francisco do better than those of driving cities like Los Angeles and Atlanta. And one of my favourite studies shows that dog owners are healthier than cat owners, presumably due to their daily walks.

My purpose with Step 2 of the South Beach Heart Programme is to give you exercise tools that are practical and can be sustained for the long-term. As with the South Beach Diet, my goal for exercise is to make it a lifestyle.

Starting at Zero

Even if you have been completely sedentary, you will reap great heart benefits by simply getting small amounts of exercise. Studies show that going from zero exercise to some exercise provides you with a greater reduction in your risk of a heart attack or stroke than going from some exercise to higher levels. Data collected from the Cooper Clinic in Dallas over a 9-year period showed that people who were sedentary had death rates that were two to three times higher than those who were moderately fit, a goal that can be achieved by walking at a comfortable pace for just 30 minutes a day, five to seven days a week. In fact, the study showed that exercise is so protective that fit people who smoked or had high blood pressure or high cholesterol had lower death rates than sedentary people who didn't smoke and had normal blood pressure and cholesterol levels. I certainly do not advocate smoking, but this study makes a strong point.

Not surprisingly, losing weight can help you go from inactive to active, practically overnight. My staff and I have found that many of our patients who lose weight on the South Beach Diet develop a desire to exercise. The reasons are varied. Some say that losing weight improved their self-esteem and inspired them to take on other challenges. Others say they felt more energetic, less encumbered, or had less joint pain. Patients who hadn't exercised for decades tell us, 'All of a sudden, I just have to move.' Whatever the reason, it's a good thing.

More Is Better

If you are already getting some exercise, I encourage you to gradually get more if you want to really help your heart. The more active you become, the more your heart and other organs benefit. As the level and intensity of your exercise routine increase, your bad LDL goes down, your good HDL goes up, and you begin to have healthy changes in the size of your LDL particles. Moderate-intensity exercise also reduces your belly fat, adds lean muscle, lowers the blood–clotting protein fibrinogen, reduces blood levels of harmful C–reactive protein, and increases your sensitivity to insulin. Doesn't all this make you want to get up off the couch right now?

A WORD OF CAUTION

Talk with your doctor before you make a sudden change in your level of activity, especially if you are aged 50 or older, have been inactive, have difficulty keeping your balance, have periods of dizziness, or have known heart problems. If you are recovering from a cardiac event, I recommend supervised cardiac rehabilitation.

People get into trouble by doing exercise they have not trained for and are not used to. The heart attack that occurs while shovelling snow is a classic case. It's not that shovelling snow is bad; in fact, as a regular exercise routine, it would be great. The problem comes when you suddenly overtax your untrained body. Overexertion when you're not fit creates a huge pulse of adrenaline that can induce a heart attack or even sudden death.

This could happen on the tennis court if you're used to playing doubles and unexpectedly get into a competitive singles match on a hot, humid day. Or it could happen at the company softball game, when you suddenly sprint to first base or slide into second. It's not that running and sliding are so bad, it's just that you have to be trained for it.

So do talk with your doctor before grabbing that snow shovel or jumping on that treadmill. Getting fit should be a gradual and careful process.

The South Beach
Heart Workout

The South Beach Heart Workout is a two-part exercise programme that features aerobic walking and a series of core-strengthening functional fitness exercises that I call the *Core Curriculum*. Doing both the walking and the core exercises should take less than an hour, but you can adapt the routine to fit any schedule. If you are new to exercising, start slowly and go at a comfortable pace. If you are already in good shape, you can move straight into the full programme. If you can only find 10 minutes to exercise, then make sure to at least get in a brisk walk.

The South Beach Heart Workout:
Aerobic Walking

Whether you've been completely sedentary or are already doing some form of aerobic exercise, I urge you to take up walking. What I recommend for most of my patients is a brisk 30-minute walk every day or most days of the week.

Aerobic exercise is essential for a healthy heart. When you start walking at the right level of intensity – or do any other vigorous low-impact aerobic activity such as swimming or bike riding – and ideally sustain that level of intensity for at least 20 minutes, you will begin to see improvements in your cholesterol and other blood fats and in your blood pressure, and you'll boost your feel-good hormones too.

One of the best things about walking is that it is natural and much easier on your joints than jogging. You can also do it anytime, anywhere. When the weather is inclement, you can do your walk at an indoor track or even in a shopping centre. Or if you want to invest in a piece of home equipment or a gym membership, you can walk on a treadmill or an elliptical trainer. Furthermore, with every step you take, you are supporting your body weight by holding yourself upright, which forces you to engage your core muscles, improving posture, stability and balance.

Getting Started

If you have been inactive and have your doctor's approval to begin a programme of brisk walking, I recommend that you start by opening your front door and walking as far as you can without feeling fatigued or stressed, even if it's for only a few minutes. Then, you can gradually increase your walking time by 2 to 5 minutes a day until you can walk briskly for 30 minutes without discomfort. In a few weeks, a 5-minute amble can become a half-hour brisk walk, giving you the level of exercise you need to begin making a lifesaving difference.

If you are already active, then I recommend that you move straight to the 30-minute brisk walk I recommend below.

Getting Up to Speed

But what exactly is a 'brisk' walk? To make things simple, I tell my patients to think of a scale of 1 to 10, with 1 being the slowest speed you can possibly walk and still keep moving and 10 being the fastest you can walk without getting out of breath. To walk 'briskly', you should be going at a pace in the 6 to 7 range, which means you're working hard, but not exhausting yourself. Try to work up a light sweat – that is a good way to gauge whether you are working hard enough. (You can also use your target heart rate to determine the correct level of exertion for you. See page 177 for how to figure it out.)

The 30-Minute Brisk Walk

Begin your walk by gradually easing into it, walking at a moderate pace to give your muscles – including your heart muscle – some time to warm up. As you walk, your muscles contract and your heart begins to pump harder to send blood to the working muscles. This raises your body temperature and prepares your muscles for increased activity. If you don't warm up your muscles before working them, they will not be as flexible and will be more prone to injury.

End your walk by gradually easing out of it, walking at a moderate pace to give your muscles time to cool down. Slowing down gradually also helps ease your heart back into normal activity.

Here's how the 30-minute walk breaks down:

5-minute warmup: Walk at an intensity level of 3 to 4 for the first 3 to 4 minutes. Work up to a pace of 6 to 7 during the last minute of the warmup.

20-minute walk: Continue at a brisk pace of 6 to 7 for 20 minutes.

5-minute cool down: For the last 5 minutes of your walk, reduce your speed to a level of 3 to 4 again. Take a few deep breaths before stopping. You should feel both relaxed and invigorated.

Don't get complacent and stay at the 6 to 7 level. As you get more fit and are able to walk without tiring, you should be increasing the intensity of your workout to the 8 to 10 range. Be sure you're not out of breath at 10, however, and that you can still carry on a conversation, even at the fastest pace.

Reaching Your Target Heart Rate

Another way to figure out whether you're walking at a brisk enough pace to improve your cardiovascular system is to see if you're reaching your target heart rate for aerobic fitness, which is about 60 per cent of your maximum heart rate (MHR).

For men: To calculate your MHR, subtract your age from 220. If you are 43, for example, your MHR is 220 - 43, or 177. If you are 58, it is 162. Multiply this resulting number by 0.60, and you will find your target heart rate, the recommended number of heartbeats per minute for improving your cardiovascular health. So, if your MHR is 177, your target heart rate is 177 x 0.60 = 106. If your MHR is 162, it's 97.

For women: To calculate your MHR, subtract your age from 226. If you are 43, for example, your MHR is 226 - 43, or 183. If you are 58, it is 168. Multiply this resulting number by 0.60, and you will find your target heart rate, the recommended number of heartbeats per minute for improving your cardiovascular health. So if your MHR is 183, your target heart rate is 183 x 0.60 = 110. If your MHR is 168, it's 101.

Now that you know the number you're aiming for, all you have to do is check your pulse when you're walking to see if you're there. To do this, you can wear a heart-rate monitor, or you can place your index finger on the side of your neck between the middle of your collarbone and your jawline (or on the radial artery on the underside of your wrist) and count the beats for 10 seconds, then multiply by 6.

If you are taking a medication such as a beta-blocker or calcium channel blocker to lower your blood pressure, be aware that certain medicines such as these may keep your heart rate lower than normal during exercise. The trick is not to overdo it; instead, make an effort to work at a moderate level of exertion. If you're taking a diuretic, be sure to drink plenty of water before exercise.

BEYOND SPEED: GETTING THE MOST OUT OF YOUR WALK

Here are some tips on how to get the most out of your walking programme.

- Pay close attention to your posture while you are walking. Keep your abdominals drawn in as you move, and consciously try to keep your belly from touching the waistband of your trousers.

- Keep your chest lifted, and imagine that your head is a helium balloon attached to a string (your spine). Your chin should stay parallel to the ground as you walk (believe it or not, leading with your chin while walking can lead to back pain). You should feel a lengthening, upright sensation throughout your body. Your muscles should not feel tense. Get into a good walking rhythm.

- With each step, strike the ground from heel to toe and feel your buttocks (glutes) contracting as you do so. This will help tone your bottom and the back of your legs as you walk.

How Fit Are You Really?

A true indication of fitness is how fast your heart can recover after you have completed your cardiovascular workout. Why is this important? It will show you how quickly your heart rate can return to normal when it is faced with a sudden challenge, such as running for a bus or having to climb a steep flight of stairs, which is not uncommon in daily life.

How do you measure your recovery rate? It's very simple. Take your pulse before beginning your walk, and make a mental note of the number of times your heart beats per minute. Immediately after finishing your walk, retake your pulse. It should be a lot higher than it was initially. Wait 90 seconds and take it again. The faster your pulse drops to where it was before you began exercising, the greater your degree of cardio fitness. If you are consistent with your walking programme, you will notice a steady but gradual improvement in your recovery time, a sign that you are increasing your cardiac endurance and strength.

Staying Motivated

Few people exercise consistently if they don't like what they're doing. To make walking (or jogging) more fun, try listening to music. Not only will it make the time pass faster and possibly improve your pace, it's actually a clinically proven motivator. In a recent study, 41 overweight women were asked to walk 2 miles 3 or more days a week. Half of the women listened to music as they walked; the other half did not. At the end of 6 months, the women who listened to music had gone for many more walks. As a result, they lost twice as much weight as the non-music group – an average of 7 kg (16 lb).

If music doesn't inspire you, find a buddy to walk with – even if it's your dog. Having a dog can force you to get out and walk, even in the rain or snow. According to a study by the Research Center for Human-Animal Interaction in Columbia, Missouri, sedentary and overweight volunteers who began walking a dog for 20 minutes a day, 5 days a week, lost an average of 6 kg (14 lb) in 1 year. Another study, published in the April 2006 issue of *Preventing Chronic Disease*, found that 80 per cent of people who take their dog for a walk get in at least one 10-minute walk a day, and 42 per cent walk 30 minutes or more. So get a dog!

If you are a digital junkie like I am, you might keep a computer record of your workout progress. Documenting your efforts and graphing your improvement is reinforcing and satisfying.

Pressed for Time?

If you don't have time to work in 30 straight minutes of walking, divide your walk into two 15-minute segments or even three 10-minute strolls. If you don't even have time for that, remember that every step counts, whether it's walking from your parked car to your office or from your desk to the coffee machine.

The South Beach Heart Workout: Core Curriculum

In addition to improving your cardiovascular system with aerobic walking (or some other cardiovascular exercise), you also need to add a regime of stretching and strengthening exercises to utilize all the different muscle groups in your body and promote functional fitness. While the exercises in my programme focus primarily on the core muscles of your abdomen, lower back, pelvis and hips, they actually help keep all your muscles and joints strong, flexible, stable and free from injury. This will enable you to live an active, heart-healthy lifestyle.

The exercises in the Core Curriculum are based on Pilates, a unique method of body conditioning developed more than 70 years ago by Joseph Pilates, a German immigrant. These exercises not only integrate stretching for enhanced flexibility, strength training focused on the core muscles, and balance, they also emphasize proper breathing and body awareness. All of the exercises are low impact and partially weight bearing, and most of them are performed in a standing or reclining position. For these reasons, they are suitable for older exercisers and people at all levels of fitness.

You may wonder how it's possible to strengthen muscles without weights. In the Core Curriculum workout, you create your own resistance by tightening your muscles and moving slowly and deliberately through each exercise. *Your body is the weight.* Furthermore, to really do these exercises properly, you need to engage both your muscles and your mind – that is, you have to concentrate on doing them correctly.

I just want to add that in addition to recommending core functional fitness as part of my heart-health programme, I also often recommend it as a way to prevent and relieve back pain. As I mentioned earlier, it is common for my patients to complain of back pain, and they often claim they can't exercise because of it. This lack of physical activity can further increase their risk of heart attack and stroke. I'm glad to see that experts in back pain are moving away from the standard back exercises and encouraging core strengthening.

Getting Started

The first and most important step in any exercise programme is to make the commitment to stick with it. Consistency is the key to success. I promise you, once you get into the exercise habit, you won't want to go back to your sedentary life.

I have found that what works best for many of my patients is to set aside a specific time every day (or every other day) to do the workout. Pick a time that you are likely to adhere to. If you're not a morning person, it's unlikely that you're going to drag yourself out of bed and onto the mat at 6 a.m., but you may actually enjoy exercising after work or in the early evening. If you find that you've missed two exercise 'appointments' because other things have come up, do some soul searching. Either you picked a time that doesn't really work for you or you're going out of your way not to exercise.

Many of the exercises described on the following pages are to be done lying on the floor, which can be a bit uncomfortable. Therefore, I suggest that you use an exercise mat or a thick towel. Do your workout in pleasant surroundings. Pick one place in your home as your exercise area and reserve it. You don't need much space, but you do need enough room to comfortably execute the exercises without bumping into furniture or having things fall on you. Be sure to wear nonbinding, comfortable clothing that allows for a full range of motion. Keep a bottle of water handy, and take a few sips between exercises if you need it. I don't recommend doing your workout in front of the television because you should focus on what you're doing. Listening to music is fine, however.

For those of you unfamiliar with exercise jargon, let me define a few terms. One repetition, or *rep*, is one complete exercise. For example, the first exercise you do is called Biceps Curls. One Biceps Curl is 1 repetition. When you do 12 repetitions, it is called a set. The goal for most of these exercises is to do three sets of 12 repetitions. In some cases, depending on the exercise, I will tell you to do more or fewer reps.

For some of you, especially those of you who haven't been doing any exercise recently, three sets of 12 repetitions may be too strenuous. On the other hand, the fit among you may find that doing three sets is too easy. In either case, do as many reps as you can without feeling pain or undue discomfort. Try to do a few more each time you work out, and you will see that over time you will improve.

Don't rush through your workout so you can fit it all in. Keep the movements fluid, flowing from one into the next. Don't rest between sets or exercises unless you feel you have to.

Those of you who have worked out before may wonder why I don't require you to 'warm up' before starting the Core Curriculum exercises. Warming up means doing something aerobic (like walking fast or bicycling) to increase your heart rate and get the blood flowing to your muscles. This helps prevent injury and is usually necessary before working out. In the case of the Core Curriculum, however, the exercises themselves are the warmup. In fact, the first group of exercises – the Arm Series – is done standing up and provides enough of a warmup that you don't need to do anything else.

As far as stretching goes, all of these exercises have a built-in stretching component. I do include two very specific stretches – the Child's Pose and the Cat 'n' Hammock Back Combination Stretch – at the end of the routine, but you will already have done plenty of stretching just by doing all of these exercises in sequence.

The Core Curriculum Exercises

Arm Series: You don't need weights or fancy gym equipment to strengthen, sculpt and tone your arms. A simple hand towel will do. The trick is to hold the towel firmly between your hands, as taut as possible. Imagine that you're trying to rip the towel apart right in the middle. If you have problems with either of your elbows (such as tennis elbow or golf elbow), don't pull so hard on the towel that it causes pain.

Do these movements slowly, keeping the towel taut. Don't forget to breathe throughout each movement. These are powerful exercises that strengthen, stretch and improve arm and shoulder function, making it easier for you to hold a child, carry a package, put a suitcase in the overhead compartment of an aeroplane, or grab a dish from the highest shelf in your kitchen.

Pelvic Bridges: These exercises help keep your spinal column supple and release any tightness in your lower back. They also help shape and tone your legs and buttocks.

Abdominal Series: These exercises are great for strengthening the entire abdominal region as well as keeping your hip joints supple.

Super Swim Exercises: Many of us spend a great deal of time hunched over in front of a computer or slumped behind the wheel of a car. These exercises, which simulate swimming, will help improve your posture by forcing you to engage back muscles that often go underused. You should only do 5 to 10 repetitions per exercise, depending on your strength. Try to work your way up to the full 10 repetitions.

Side Toners: These exercises improve spinal, pelvis and shoulder alignment and connection. They also improve balance and abdominal strength.

Stretch It Out: You've just worked your lower back, so now you need to release your lower-back muscles by doing these two stretches – the Child's Pose and the Cat 'n' Hammock Back Combination Stretch.

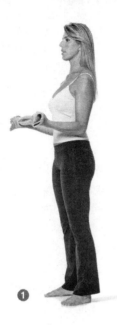 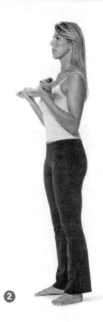

BICEPS CURLS

1. Stand with your legs shoulder-width apart and your feet flat on the floor. Keep both feet directly below your knees for better stability. Grasp a hand towel firmly with both hands, palms up. Keeping your elbows tightly at your sides, raise your forearms until they're at about a 90-degree angle to your waist. Make sure that your wrists and elbows are in a straight line in front of you. Try as hard as you can to pull the towel apart.

2. As you keep pulling, lift the towel to your chest to a count of 1, 2, 3 and then lower it to your thighs to a count of 1, 2, 3. Keep the tension on the towel as you lift it up and down. Try to imagine that you are lifting a heavy weight. This should be a fluid up-and-down movement, with no stopping between repetitions. Keep working against resistance, as if one arm is fighting the other to hold onto the towel. If you feel like you're working hard, it's because you are. Work your way up to three sets of 12 repetitions.

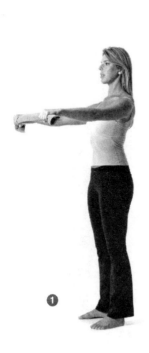

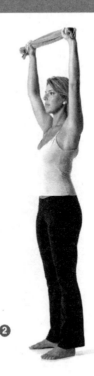

ARM RAISES

1. Stand with your legs shoulder-width apart and your feet flat on the floor. Keep both feet directly below your knees for better stability. Grasp a hand towel firmly with both hands, palms down. Extend your arms straight out in front of you at about chest level, shoulder-width apart. Keep your elbows and wrists in a straight line. Try as hard as you can to pull the towel apart.

2. As you keep pulling, lift your arms as high as you comfortably can to a count of 1, 2, 3. (The goal is to try to lift your arms over your head.) Then bring your arms back down to thigh height to a count of 1, 2, 3. Keep the tension on the towel as you lift it up and down. Try to imagine that you are lifting a heavy weight. This should be a fluid movement with no stopping between repetitions. Work your way up to three sets of 12 reps.

Caution: Stop if you feel any shoulder pain as you lift your arms overhead.

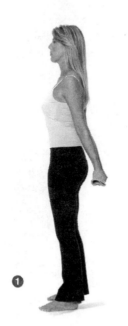
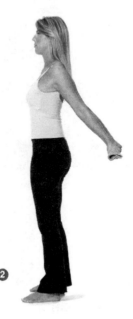

TRICEPS PULLS

1. Stand with your legs shoulder-width apart and your feet flat on the floor. Keep both feet directly below your knees for better stability. Grab a hand towel behind your bottom with both palms facing forwards.

2. Try as hard as you can to pull the towel apart. Keep your shoulder blades pinched as you raise the towel up and away from your bottom as high as you can to a count of 1, 2, 3. Be sure to keep your arms straight, your abdominals pulled in, and your chest lifted; don't allow your back to sway. Then lower the towel back to your bottom to a count of 1, 2, 3. This should be a fluid up-and-down movement, with no stopping between repetitions. Work your way up to three sets of 12 reps.

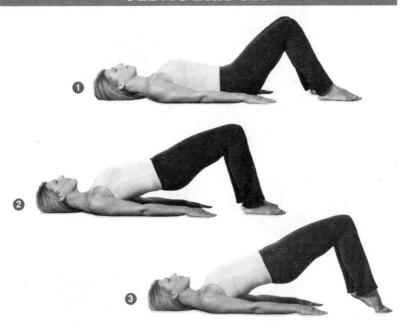

BASIC BRIDGE AND LIFTED HEEL BRIDGE VARIATION

If you have difficulty doing the Basic Bridge, skip the Lifted Heel Bridge Variation (Step 3) until you have mastered the Basic Bridge.

1. Lie on your back with your arms at your sides and your knees bent. Keep your knees shoulder-width apart and press your feet firmly into the floor. Press your shoulder blades into the floor and feel your chest softening.

2. Starting at your tailbone, gently and slowly lift your back off the floor up to your shoulder blades. Once you reach this position, tighten your abdominal muscles to support your spine. Squeeze your buttock muscles tightly and hold for a count of 10 while keeping your pelvis lifted evenly (pretend you have to balance a cup of hot tea on it!). After a count of 10, slowly roll your spine back to the floor, one vertebra at a time. Work up to three sets of 12 repetitions.

3. When you've mastered the Basic Bridge, try the Lifted Heel Bridge Variation. Repeat the Basic Bridge, but as you lift your back off the floor also lift your heels off the floor. Keep them elevated until you roll your entire spine back to the floor. This gives your lower body and feet an even better stretch.

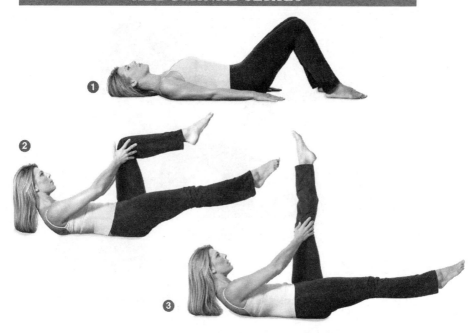

ALTERNATING KNEE PULL AND STRAIGHT LEG PULL VARIATION

1. Lie on your back with your arms at your sides and your knees bent. Keep your knees shoulder-width apart and press your feet firmly into the floor.

2. Lift your head and the top of your shoulder blades off the floor using your abdominal muscles, not your neck muscles. (If you feel any strain on your neck, you are not lifting properly from your abdomen.) Place both of your hands just below one knee and pull the knee towards your chest. As you do so, extend your other leg, holding it about 30 cm (1 ft) off the floor. While keeping your abdominal muscles tight and without lowering your head or your legs to the floor, switch legs. Continue to switch legs, keeping the transition from one leg to the other smooth. Gradually increase your pace, but keep the movements fluid. Work up to three sets of 12 repetitions.

3. Once you have mastered the Alternating Knee Pull, you can try the Straight Leg Pull Variation, which is more challenging. Lie on your back with your knees bent, your arms at your sides, and your head raised off the floor, as it is in Step 2. Straighten one leg, place your hands behind the knee, and gently pull it towards your chest. At the same time, straighten your other leg, and raise and hold it about 30 cm (1 ft) off the ground. While keeping your abdominal muscles tight and without lowering your head or your legs to the floor, switch legs. Continue to switch legs, keeping the transition from one leg to the other smooth. Gradually increase your pace, but keep the movements fluid. Work up to three sets of 12 repetitions.

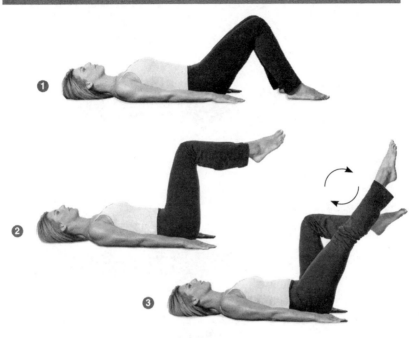

BICYCLE

1. Lie on your back with your arms by your sides and your knees bent. Keep your knees shoulder-width apart and press your feet firmly into the floor. Tightly squeeze your abdominal muscles.

2. Keeping your abdominals tight, raise both legs off the ground so that your knees are at a 90-degree angle to your hips. (If you can't get to 90 degrees, do what feels good.)

3. Pretend you are on a bicycle, and begin peddling your legs in the air. Be sure to keep your abdominal muscles tight and your back pressed into the floor so you don't strain your lower back. Peddle forwards 12 times and then switch directions and peddle backwards 12 times. For this exercise, one complete set is equal to 12 forward peddles and 12 backward peddles. Work up to three sets of 12 forward and 12 backward repetitions.

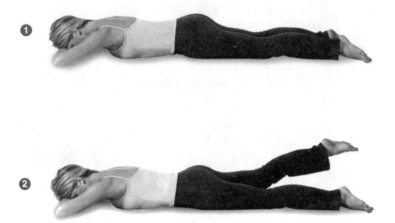

SINGLE LEG LIFT, DOUBLE LEG LIFT VARIATION AND HEEL BEAT VARIATION

1. Lie facedown with your forehead on the backs of your hands. Tighten your abdominal and buttock muscles, and try to create a space between your belly button and the floor. (Keeping your abdominal and buttock muscles tight as you do this will help prevent back strain.)

2. Point your toes and lift one leg off the floor as high as you can without straining your back. Hold the leg in that position for a count of 1, 2. Lower the leg to the floor, then repeat with the other leg for a count of 1, 2. Work up to three sets of 5 to 10 repetitions.

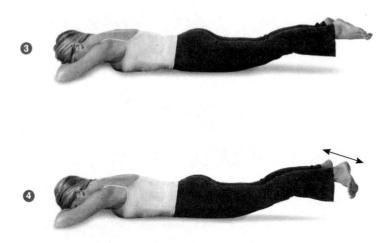

3. Once you have mastered the Single Leg Lift, you can try the Double Leg Lift Variation, which is more challenging. Follow Step 1, then proceed as follows: point your toes, then lift both legs off the floor as high as you can without straining your back. Hold your legs in this position for a count of 10. Lower your legs to the floor and repeat. Work up to three sets of 5 to 10 repetitions.

4. Once you have mastered the Double Leg Lift Variation, you can try the Heel Beat Variation, which is even more challenging. Follow Step 1 (opposite page), then proceed as follows: lift both legs as high as you can off the floor without straining your back. Flex both feet while holding your legs about 15 cm (6 in) apart at the ankles. Open and close your legs quickly to a count of 30 beats (don't allow your heels to touch). In this exercise, 30 beats is 1 repetition. Work up to three sets of 30 beats each.

Caution: *Stop the exercise if you feel any discomfort in your back.*

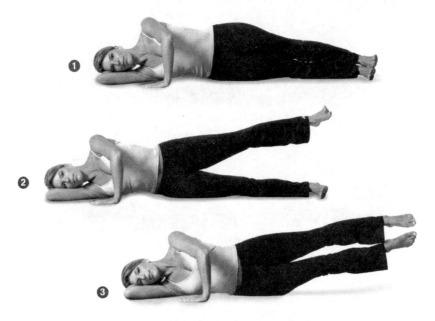

TOP LEG LIFT AND LOWER LEG LIFT VARIATION

1. Lie on your right side with your right arm folded under your ear and your left arm in front of you, palm down by your right shoulder. Your hips and shoulders should be aligned top and bottom. Tighten your abdominal muscles. Use your forward hand for leverage, and try to lift your waist off the floor.

2. Keeping your abdominals tight, lift your top leg to hip height as you press your bottom leg into the floor to improve your stability. Keep your hips and shoulders aligned, and don't allow them to roll forwards. Work the outer thigh as you slowly lift and lower the top leg in one continuous motion. As you lift and lower your leg, pretend that there is a weight on top of your thigh that you are resisting. After completing as many repetitions as you can, roll over and repeat on the other side. Work up to three sets of 12 repetitions for each leg.

3. Once you've mastered the Top Leg Lift, you can try the Lower Leg Lift Variation, which is more challenging. Follow Step 1 above and then proceed as follows: keeping your abdominals tight, lift your top leg to hip height and hold it there. Lift your bottom leg to touch the anklebone of the top leg, then slowly lower the bottom leg back to the floor. Keep your top leg in place as you lift and lower your bottom leg. Keep the movement going, and don't stop between repetitions. After completing as many lifts as you can, roll over and repeat on the other side. Work up to three sets of 12 repetitions for each leg.

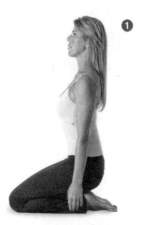

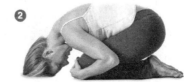

CHILD'S POSE

1. Kneel on the floor with your knees and feet together. Sit on your heels, keeping your arms by your sides with your palms facing inwards.

2. Pull your abdominals towards your spine, round your back, and lean forwards, bringing your head forwards and downwards as far as you can. Don't force the movement. You should feel a stretch throughout your entire back. Hold this position for 30 seconds and return to the upright position. Repeat the stretch 3 to 5 times.

   Caution: Stop this exercise if you experience knee pain.

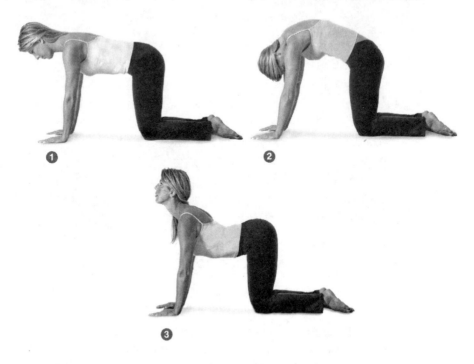

① ② ③

CAT 'N' HAMMOCK BACK COMBINATION STRETCH

This combination of two easy stretches improves spine flexibility and strengthens the abdominal muscles.

1. Get on your hands and knees with your back in a flat, tabletop position. Your hands should be in line with your shoulders and your knees in line with your hips.

2. Press your palms into the floor and pull your abdominal muscles towards your spine. Squeeze your buttock muscles and arch your back and neck like a cat. Hold this position for 10 seconds.

3. From the Cat Stretch, flow into the Hammock Back Stretch. Pull your shoulders down and away from your ears and slowly raise your head. Keeping your abdominal muscles tight, allow your back to sway down as if you were a human hammock. Hold this position for 10 seconds, then return to the flat back position. Alternate in a flowing manner between the Cat Stretch and the Hammock Back Stretch 3 to 5 times. End with the Cat Stretch.

Jane's Story

'Exercise has changed my life.'

I've been chubby and slow-moving most of my life. When I was a child, I had a book called *The Poky Little Puppy,* which was about a puppy who was always slower than the rest of the pack. That was me. I had no interest in moving fast or doing sports of any kind. As a result, I wore 'chubby' sizes when I was in primary school and adult sizes when I was in secondary school. I just didn't move.

When I reached middle age, I was not getting exercise of any kind and I was wearing 'plus' sizes. Some people are twitchers and fidgeters. I could sit for hours without moving a muscle. If I had to get out of a chair, it took mental effort. It's not surprising that I weighed 122 kg (19 st 3 lb) by the time I was 50. I wasn't a binge eater, and I never gained a lot of weight at any given time. I just added a couple of pounds a year. Do that for 40 years, and you're 36 kg (5 st 7 lb) pounds overweight.

I went in for a long-overdue medical 2 years ago. I was surprised to find out that I had high blood sugar, borderline high blood pressure and high LDL cholesterol. But I didn't do anything about my health until my husband developed high blood pressure and was told to go on an exercise programme. He really wanted me to join him. I agreed to do it for a few weeks just to get him involved. To my surprise, I found that after a few weeks, I was actually enjoying the walks we took together.

Now, a year later, I've lost almost 23 kg (3½ st) and look and feel very different. I'm out of plus sizes and have had to replace my entire wardrobe. I can go into any department store and find clothes that fit. My husband and I still go for walks most days of the week. My cholesterol is down and my blood sugar is normal. I also have a lot more energy. On some days, a morning walk doesn't feel like enough exercise to me, so I'll go for another walk in the afternoon. I can be on the go all day and not be tired. I've gone from someone who didn't want to move at all to someone who looks for ways to get more exercise. I had no idea this could happen to anyone, much less me. Exercise has changed my life. I know now that you just have to get started. ■

STEP
3

GETTING THE RIGHT
DIAGNOSTIC TESTS

Doctors now have the diagnostic tools to detect cardiovascular disease in its earliest stages, years if not decades before a heart attack or stroke occurs. Unfortunately, too few people are taking advantage of these tools. For this reason, I encourage you to read this part of the programme and discuss what you learn with your doctor. It describes the most up-to-date tests for predicting whether you're a candidate for a heart attack or stroke, as well as the appropriate follow-up tests.

Although the sophisticated tests reviewed here are becoming more widely used, some, including EBT and advanced lipoprotein testing, are not generally available in the UK on the NHS and may not be covered by private health insurance either. I would recommend discussing these questions with your GP with a view to referral to a prevention-oriented doctor or cardiologist. Cardiac CT is available in some specialist centres in the UK. It is essential that an experienced radiologist or cardiologist conducts the test to ensure its accuracy and correct interpretation.

Why These Tests Are Needed

It's critical to remember that a healthy percentage of all heart attacks occur in people who have *none* or *one* of the obvious risk factors for heart disease. These men and women don't smoke, they don't have a bad family history, and even their total cholesterol and LDL and HDL cholesterol levels may be fine by conventional laboratory standards.

Some cardiac risk factors can *only* be detected through the more sophisticated diagnostic tests explained here. For example, getting advanced blood testing is the only way to find out the size and density of your LDL particles, whether your HDL is the right size, or if you have high levels of lipoprotein (a). As I discussed in Chapter 4, many individuals whose numbers look normal on a Standard Lipid Profile may nevertheless be building up plaque and harbouring these potentially dangerous cholesterol particles. Without advanced blood testing, these people would never know they are at risk for a heart attack.

I realize that Step 3 involves getting diagnostic tests that are not usually available on the NHS and may not even be covered by many private health insurance schemes. But to really assess your level of risk for heart disease, you must go beyond conventional testing, even if it means investing some of your own money. While a noninvasive angiogram (heart scan) can cost about £800, you can get your Calcium Score alone for about £400. Advanced blood testing may be covered by insurance, but can cost an extra couple of hundred pounds. I realize that some of you may be dismayed by the prospect of having to pay more. However, I believe that getting these tests is one of the best investments you will ever make.

In My Office

When I see a new patient in my practice, I first take a complete medical history and do a physical exam. As a preventive cardiologist, I focus on the person's cardiac history and cardiac risk factors. If there is a strong family history of heart disease as well as several other cardiac risk factors, I go right into an aggressive prevention mode. In other words, I strongly advise these patients to get advanced as well as routine blood testing and a heart scan. In patients with a mixed picture of cardiac risk, I still recommend a heart scan to better assess their true cardiac risk.

Even with those patients at seemingly low risk for a heart attack or stroke, I frankly discuss the potential benefits of advanced testing. I tell these patients that while I am fairly confident that they are at low risk, this does not mean *no* risk. They could still be building up substantial plaque in their coronary arteries and heading for a heart attack. I also tell them that having further testing is totally up to them. If they do want to go ahead, I suggest that they begin with advanced blood testing and then, if the blood test indicates hidden risk, we can have another discussion about the importance of a heart scan.

Having images of a patient's coronary arteries from a heart scan greatly helps the patient understand what has to be done next. When patients see the buildup of plaque in their own coronary arteries, they are much more likely to be diligent about watching their diet, getting more exercise and taking their medications.

One interesting scenario I commonly see in my practice illustrates this point very well. A wife will literally drag her overweight and sedentary husband into the office because she believes he is at risk for heart disease. She wants me to 'read him the riot act'. If, after taking a history and doing the appropriate tests, I find he truly is at high risk, I will definitely read him the riot act. I don't let a patient like this leave the office until he fully understands that unless he takes action, he is putting his life in jeopardy.

Sometimes, however, the tests show that even though the husband is carrying extra weight and never exercises, he is not at high risk for a heart attack or stroke. Even when this is true, I still encourage lifestyle changes and explain the reasons why they are important. To the consternation of the wife, who was anticipating more radical measures, I am not as forceful as I would be with a high-risk patient. I give this patient the best information I can, but, ultimately, compliance is up to him.

Sometimes, however, the wife doesn't give up. In future visits, I often observe what my nurses and I call the 'Yes, Yes, No, No' sign.

Upon the couple's return, I ask the husband, 'Have you started your exercise programme?' or 'Have you stopped smoking?' While he nods his head 'yes, yes', his spouse is vigorously shaking her head 'no, no'. Again, the best I can do is to try to get the husband to understand his risks and the reasoning behind my recommendations. Most importantly, I also let him know that I will work with him even if he isn't willing to do everything I say. He just needs to be willing to do *something*. Even making small changes can reduce the risk of having a heart attack or stroke. And those small changes often lead to bigger ones.

My goal in Step 3 is to provide you with the information you need to open a dialogue with your doctor. *Remember, when it comes to heart disease, it's what you don't know that can kill you.* If you get the preventive tests I recommend, you will find out if you are at risk, you will be able to get the aggressive treatment required, and hopefully you will prevent a heart attack or stroke. This goal is being accomplished in more and more doctors' surgeries around the country.

In the pages that follow, I describe an annual exam and provide explanations of the discretionary diagnostic laboratory tests I recommend. While my recommendations vary from patient to patient depending on age, risk factors and the person's attitude toward treatment, this basic information nevertheless will help you decide with your own doctor what tests are best for you.

An Annual Medical Examination

If you don't have an annual medical examination, you should. This is an opportunity to evaluate your risk of a heart attack or stroke early, while there is plenty of time to do something about it.

When you visit your doctor, you should bring up anything that has affected your lifestyle, such as a change in your ability to exercise. I always want to know about patients' exercise habits and how long and how hard they can exercise comfortably. This is called *exercise tolerance* or *exercise capacity*, and it is especially important in helping me assess their heart health.

I often tell patients that daily exercise not only provides direct health benefits but is also a useful diagnostic tool. For example, almost everyone experiences some kind of chest discomfort or shortness of breath from time to time. If a patient tells me they're panting on the treadmill and can't do their usual exercise routine (in other words, their exercise capacity has definitely decreased), I become concerned and will likely do an exercise stress test (see pages 212–14) to further evaluate their symptoms. But if the person's symptoms do not affect his or her ability to walk or jog as usual, then I am less concerned. One example of this is the feeling of 'air hunger' people often experience when they can't seem to get a deep breath. When this happens, most people get panicky, start hyperventilating, and their symptoms only worsen. This type of shortness of breath is characteristically not brought on by exercise. We call this a 'sighing' respiratory pattern, and it usually represents neither heart nor lung problems.

The reason I bring all this up is to point out that if you are making your first visit to a new doctor, you will want to be prepared with as much relevant history as possible. This will save you and your doctor time and make your visit more productive. If you sense that a doctor has less time for you than you'd like, you are undoubtedly right; most GPs have external stresses on their practices that force them to have less time for you these days. Therefore, the more knowledgeable and focused you are when you arrive at the surgery, the better and the more productive your relationship with your doctor will be.

In addition to discussing lifestyle factors such as exercise and diet with your doctor, be prepared to talk about your cardiac risk factors, including your family history. It is also important to bring a list of your medications, including the dosages you are taking (check the bottles' labels) and when and how often you take the medications (once or twice daily, with meals, and so on). The list should also include any drugs you cannot take due to ineffectiveness or adverse reactions, including allergy. It is frustrating when new patients come into my office and say they are on a medication for high blood pressure or high cholesterol, but they don't know the name or the dosage. (Also remember to include supplements.)

Another way to save you and your doctor some time is to write down the dates of medical events in your history, such as hospitalizations and previous surgeries, and bring that with you as well.

Once you've given your doctor your history and discussed any particular health problems you may be experiencing, you will have your vital signs taken and be examined. Your doctor may order a number of routine tests, including a complete blood count, a chemistry profile that includes liver and kidney function, a blood sugar (glucose) test, a Standard Lipid Profile to check your blood fats, and an electrocardiogram (ECG) to show the heart's rhythm. Since the Standard Lipid Profile and ECG can provide key information about your heart health, I have included information about them here.

The Standard Lipid Profile

What is it? A measure of the levels of various blood fats (or *lipids*), the Standard Lipid Profile (also known as a *complete lipid profile*) is the most basic laboratory blood test done in doctors' surgeries to evaluate cardiac risk. It is a test in which blood is usually, though not always, drawn in the fasting state. This blood test provides a measurement of your total cholesterol, LDL ('bad') cholesterol, HDL ('good') cholesterol and triglyceride levels. It's important to note that the Standard Lipid Profile does not include a breakdown of the size of your LDL or HDL. You can only get this information by having advanced blood testing, which I describe in detail on pages 204–8.

Laboratories usually include on the printout of these measurements the normal ranges for each of the components of the lipid profile. It should be remembered that what constitutes a dangerous lipid level in one person might not be harmful for the next. Every individual lays down plaque differently, and some people with lower lipids may be more likely to have a heart attack than those with slightly higher levels. 'Normal' levels are guidelines for the general population and are not absolute for individuals. Your lipid profile should be evaluated by your doctor in the context of your own overall risk profile. As discussed in Chapter 4, for those at high risk, including patients who have sustained a heart attack, lowering what are even quite low cholesterol levels even further can prevent future heart attacks.

Joint British Societies guidelines suggest the following:

- **Total cholesterol.** Whether you're a man or a woman, your total cholesterol should be below 5 mmol/L and below 4 mmol/L for those at higher risk.

- **LDL ('bad') cholesterol.** For men and women at low risk for heart disease, LDL should be below 3 mmol/L. For those at high risk for heart disease, LDL should be less than 2 mmol/L. Most people require a prescription medication, such as a statin, to get their LDL level down this low. I describe statins and other medications in Step 4 of the South Beach Heart Programme.

- **HDL ('good') cholesterol.** An HDL level of below 1 mmol/L for men and 1.3 mmol/L for women is used to identify those with increased risk. For high-risk men and women, my goal is to achieve an HDL/LDL ratio of approximately 1 to 1. If your HDL is low, getting more exercise, taking prescription niacin and/or statin drugs, losing weight (if necessary), stopping smoking and maintaining a healthy diet can help raise it.

- **Triglycerides.** For both men and women, triglyceride levels should be below 1.7 mmol/L. For high-risk patients, my goal is a triglyceride level of less than 1.1 mmol/L. Losing weight, taking prescription niacin and fish oil supplements, and avoiding starchy and sugary carbohydrates as well as saturated fat and trans fats are all effective ways of reducing elevated levels of this bad type of blood fat. I call triglycerides and HDL *lifestyle lipids* because they are both very sensitive to changes in diet and exercise.

Follow-up. Joint British Societies recommend that full risk assessment, including Standard Lipid Profile, is performed at least every 5 years. However, for those with risk factors for heart disease and those already on lipid-lowering medications, the test should be repeated more often. Depending on a patient's level of risk, I repeat the lipid profile every 2 to 4 months until our goal is reached. I then repeat the lipid profile every 6 months along with a liver profile for those taking lipid-lowering medications, such as statins. If a change in the patient's diet or exercise routine causes that person to lose or gain weight, I repeat the lipid profile sooner.

Electrocardiogram

What is it? An electrocardiogram (ECG) is a simple, noninvasive, completely painless test that takes just minutes. It is now available in many general practices or you may be required to attend your local hospital. You lie down on an examining table and a technician applies a gel and small patches to your chest, arms and legs. The heart's electrical activity is recorded as a series of waves (*tracings*) on a strip of paper. It is important to note that a resting ECG does not reflect the electrical activity of your heart under stress. ECGs can be abnormal for many reasons. An abnormal ECG does not necessarily indicate life-threatening heart disease. Further tests will be done to clarify whether the abnormality represents a real problem.

Follow-up. It is useful to have an ECG performed routinely, so if new symptoms develop, a new ECG can be performed and compared to a recent one. If you have heart attack symptoms such as chest pain at rest while the new ECG is being taken, the new test may show problems not detected earlier, and this helps your doctor make a diagnosis more quickly. If you've never had a baseline ECG and suddenly develop chest pain, a doctor may mistake a perfectly normal variation in your heart for signs of an imminent problem and treat you more aggressively than necessary.

Discretionary Tests

At your routine evaluation, you can discuss the value of the advanced diagnostic tests described below with your GP. Your doctor may want to wait to review the results of your Standard Lipid Profile before making a determination about additional tests. If you feel strongly that you would like to have advanced blood testing or a heart scan done, discuss your reasons with your doctor or with a preventive cardiologist.

Advanced Blood Testing

What is it? Advanced blood testing includes all those tests beyond the Standard Lipid Profile that have been shown to help predict cardiac risk. This more advanced blood analysis explains why so many patients without many conventional risk factors still have heart attacks. When I first began doing heart scans, I was confused by the number of patients who had large amounts of plaque and yet still had normal levels of LDL and HDL cholesterol. When I began getting advanced blood testing on these patients, it almost always explained why the patient had accumulated plaque, and I could then figure out what I could do to slow or stop the atherosclerotic process.

I recommend the following advanced blood testing for any patients who have risk factors for coronary disease. Some of the lab work requires more sophisticated equipment than doing the Standard Lipid Profile, so it may not be available in all laboratories.

LIPOPROTEIN SUBFRACTION TEST

This is an exacting blood test that divides your cholesterol into a variety of subparticles based on their size and density. While the Standard Lipid Profile tells you the *quantity* of total cholesterol, LDL, HDL and triglycerides, this test will tell you the *quality* of your cholesterol. In particular, you will learn whether you have large amounts of small, dense LDL and/or small HDL particles, both of which put you at risk of having a heart attack or stroke.

As I discussed in Chapter 4, the rate at which cholesterol gets into your vessel walls depends on the number and size of your LDL cholesterol particles. Small LDL particles containing less cholesterol per particle move into vessel walls more easily than larger particles. The smaller the particle, the more easily it moves in. That's why patients who have low total cholesterol levels and even low total LDL levels can still be at high risk for coronary disease if they have lots of small LDL. Patients with increased numbers of small LDL particles are classified as being *pattern B*. Those with large LDL particles are classified as *pattern A*.

Like small LDL, small HDL also has less cholesterol per particle. Patients with predominantly small HDL particles do not clear cholesterol from vessel walls as well as those with larger HDL particles. Small HDL also reduces the total cholesterol number, and this is another reason why patients with low total cholesterol may still be at risk for coronary disease. That's why it is important to know not just your total cholesterol and LDL numbers, but also the size of your particles.

People who have small LDL and HDL along with high triglycerides have what is called the *atherogenic lipid profile* and must be treated aggressively. These lipid factors are associated with a sedentary lifestyle, obesity, prediabetes and diabetes – and will accelerate the development of atherosclerosis. A programme of weight loss (outlined in Step 1 of my programme) and regular exercise can help to reverse these lipid abnormalities. Taking medications such as a slow-release form of niacin (Niaspan), fenofibrate (Lipantil), or one of the so-called TZD agents, rosiglitazone maleate (Avandia) or pioglitazone hydrochloride (Actos), can also help.

LIPOPROTEIN (a) TEST

Lipoprotein (a), or Lp(a), is a type of LDL particle with a protein called 'little a' attached. An increased number of these particles is associated with an increased risk of coronary disease when Lp(a) is greater than 30 mg/dL. (This number could be slightly higher or lower depending on the lab that analyses the blood test.) This risk is multiplied when Lp(a) is associated with other blood lipid abnormalities, such as elevated LDL.

How Lp(a) actually affects your blood vessels is still not well understood, but you can think of it as making the endothelial lining of the arterial walls more porous to LDL particles. Thus, Lp(a) facilitates the development of plaque, which can lead to heart attacks. Lp(a) is unique in that it does not respond to lifestyle changes. Niacin is the only medication that effectively lowers Lp(a), though it often requires high doses.

Follow-up. When the results of the lipoprotein subclass and Lp(a) tests are abnormal, I treat a patient with lifestyle changes and medications accordingly and repeat the tests every 2 to 6 months depending on the patient's overall level of risk. Once the therapeutic goals are reached, I repeat the tests twice a year.

HIGH-SENSITIVITY C-REACTIVE PROTEIN (hs-CRP) TEST

C-reactive protein is a protein particle that is elevated when there is inflammation in the body, whether from a viral infection, a bacterial infection, arthritis or an injury, including the chronic injury to the arterial walls that is part of the atherosclerotic process. Elevated CRP is also associated with a greater tendency for the blood to clot. This makes plaque rupture more likely to produce a large enough blood clot to block bloodflow in an artery and cause a heart attack. The advanced blood test is called a high-sensitivity C-reactive protein (hs-CRP) test to differentiate it from a basic CRP test. For both men and women, the amount of CRP in the blood is a good overall predictor of the risk of having a heart attack. You are at low risk if the amount of CRP in your blood is 1 mg/L or less, at average risk if the amount is between 1 and 3 mg/L, and at high risk if your level is above 4 mg/L.

An elevated level of CRP is often found in smokers and in patients with central obesity (belly fat) and diabetes. It is also often elevated in patients with chronic periodontal disease. As I noted in Chapter 3, inflammation is associated not only with heart attack and stroke, but also with other chronic diseases of Western civilization, including cancer, Alzheimer's disease and macular degeneration.

In order to accurately tell whether a patient's elevated hs-CRP is truly a sign of chronic underlying inflammation, the test should be repeated three times with at least several weeks in between, and only when there are no apparent infections or injuries. Exercise, weight loss, smoking cessation and statin drugs help to lower hs–CRP.

Follow-up. If the hs–CRP test is normal, the test need not be repeated routinely unless there is a change in risk factors, such as weight, exercise frequency or smoking status. If it is elevated, I generally repeat the test every few months to monitor its response to favourable lifestyle changes and/or medications.

HOMOCYSTEINE TEST

Homocysteine is a product of protein metabolism and has been found to be a risk factor for heart attack, stroke and other vascular diseases. Its role as a cardiac risk factor was first brought to light by Harvard researcher Dr Kilmer McCully in 1969. Dr McCully had noticed that children with genetically inherited homocystinuria (the inability to metabolize homocysteine and other amino acids normally) developed vascular disease at very young ages. In these children, homocysteine built up to very high levels in the blood until it spilled over into the urine. Dr McCully reasoned that if extremely high homocysteine levels could cause early vascular disease, perhaps lower levels that were still higher than normal might be a risk factor for heart disease in adults. After years of scepticism, his theory has been borne out. Whether you are a man or a woman, if you have a homocysteine level of 12 µmol/L, you are at greater risk for a heart attack or stroke.

What has not been proven is whether treating high homocysteine levels with a cocktail of B vitamins (which many doctors have been recommending) can prevent heart attack and stroke in high–risk people. My suggestion is to eat plenty of whole fruits and vegetables and other foods that contain B vitamins, but avoid the supplements.

Follow-up. A yearly test for homocysteine may be helpful in reassessing risk.

HAEMOGLOBIN A1c TEST

This is a simple blood test that reflects the average level of your blood sugar over the prior 3 months. As such, it gives a more meaningful picture of what is happening with your blood sugar than an isolated blood glucose test. There isn't one number that truly divides normal from abnormal blood sugar. A haemoglobin A1c level of 5.7 per cent or higher is borderline, and greater than 7 per cent is where we begin to see complications of diabetes. Those who have gained weight in middle age and have a level close to 5.5 per cent are at risk of future diabetes if they continue to gain weight.

Follow-up. If a patient's haemoglobin A1c level is borderline or elevated, I repeat the test every 3 to 6 months to monitor the person's improvement – or lack thereof – with diet, other lifestyle changes and medications. Along with monitoring triglycerides and HDL, following haemoglobin A1c is an excellent way for both the patient and the doctor to monitor the success of their efforts.

Heart Scan

What is it? A heart scan is a noninvasive procedure that shows the amount of calcified plaque you have in your coronary arteries. Currently, two types of heart scanners are being used. The first is the multislice computed tomography (CT) scanner, which creates an extremely detailed cross-sectional image of your arteries using x-ray cameras. The second is the electron-beam tomography (EBT) scanner, which creates images of the heart using an electron gun.

Both types of scanners are excellent, and the one you choose depends on what your doctor recommends and what type of equipment is available at your hospital. It may also depend on how much money you are willing to spend. There are advantages to each.

The advantage of the EBT scanner is that it acquires images faster than a multislice scanner. This is particularly important when imaging a moving organ such as the heart. But while an EBT scan will provide an accurate Calcium Score and show the extent of your coronary disease, it cannot consistently show the presence and extent of *soft plaque*. That is the true benefit of the new, state-of-the-art 64-slice scan. Remember, it is the cholesterol-filled soft plaque that can grow, rupture and cause a heart attack, so it is good to know if there is soft plaque lurking inside the lining of your artery walls.

The 64-slice scanner is simply the latest in a long line of multislice scanners, many of which are still being used. The first multislice scanner was the 4-slice, introduced in the early 1990s. It was followed by 8-, 16-, and 32-slice scanners. Some hospitals are still using this earlier technology but, while some of these scans can give you an accurate Calcium Score, the 64-slice scan is the best at imaging soft plaque with a dye injection (as I mentioned earlier, this is called a *noninvasive angiogram*). You may have been told that the 64-slice scanner can actually *quantify* the percentage of obstruction in your arteries. While it may be able to do this in certain patients, results are often unreliable. The invasive angiogram is still the best technique for determining the *percentage* of blockage. That said, a noninvasive angiogram is useful for *excluding obstruction*. In other words, if your scan looks completely normal, you can be confident that it is accurately showing that there are no blockages.

From a patient's perspective, having a heart scan is quite easy. You lie down fully clothed on an examination table, the scanner passes over you for a minute or two, and then it's over. If a contrast dye is used, you may have to fast beforehand and the examination can take a little longer. One caveat: if you've ever had an allergic reaction to a contrast dye or iodine or have an allergy to shellfish, you should consider a scan that involves contrast dye injection only under special circumstances. Be sure to tell your doctor about any such allergies or reactions. Premedication can be used to minimize an allergic reaction to the dye. Caution must also be used in patients with compromised kidney function (often found in people with diabetes) since the dye can worsen the situation. You should also tell your doctor if you are or might be pregnant; if so, you should not have a scan at all.

Once the scanned image of your heart has been analysed, it's converted into a number ranging from 0 to several thousand. As I discussed in Chapter 6, this number is called your *Calcium Score*. The higher your score compared to others of your age and sex, the more calcified plaque you have in your arteries and the greater your risk for a future heart attack. For your convenience, here again is the chart that appeared in Chapter 6.

UNDERSTANDING YOUR CALCIUM SCORE

Calcium Score for a 55-Year-Old Man or Woman	Relative Amount of Plaque
0–10	Minimal
11–100	Moderate
101–400	Increased
401+	Extensive

As I mentioned earlier, one of the real benefits of the heart scan is that I can show my patients pictures of their actual coronary arteries and the extent of plaque buildup. It's one thing to tell patients – especially those who don't have any overt symptoms – that there's a buildup of plaque in their artery walls and that they have to take a medication and make some lifestyle changes. It's quite another to have them see their plaque firsthand (coronary calcium shows up as bright white spots on the scan). I've found that a compelling visual provides strong motivation for patients to stay on their treatment programme, and in particular to keep taking their medications. Moreover, follow-up heart scans can help you and your doctor keep track of your progress and make any necessary adjustments to your treatment programme.

Follow-up. If you have few or no calcium deposits, you need not repeat the heart scan for at least 5 years. If you do have signs of calcium buildup, the test can be repeated every 2 to 5 years, depending on your other risk factors.

Echocardiogram (Ultrasound of the Heart)

What is it? An echocardiogram, or ultrasound of the heart, is a non-invasive test that takes about 30 minutes and uses ultrasound technology to provide a picture of the structures of the heart. A water-soluble gel is applied to the skin on your chest, then the ultrasound technician places a device called a transducer on the chest wall to bounce sound waves off the walls and valves of your heart. The sound waves return to the transducer as echoes, which are then converted into sharp moving images of your beating heart and its valves as they open and close. The echocardiogram shows the size of each of the four heart chambers and the function of the major pumping chamber, the left ventricle.

Patients with damage from a heart attack or who have high blood pressure or valve problems will have abnormalities that are readily apparent on the echocardiogram. By adding Doppler ultrasound to the equipment, we get a good picture of the blood actually flowing through the heart. This allows us to assess the presence and extent of valve leaks and valve narrowing, but we cannot reliably visualize bloodflow in the coronary arteries.

For cardiac prevention, I obtain an echocardiogram in patients with high blood pressure to evaluate the thickness of the left ventricle. If blood pressure is elevated day in and day out, the heart has to push harder to eject the blood. When it does this, the heart muscle gets thicker, just as your biceps do when you are regularly lifting weights.

Walking around, it's easy to see who is spending the most time in the gym pumping iron because their muscles are bulging out of their tailored clothes. Similarly, I can tell whose heart has been pumping the hardest on a regular basis by the thickness of the left ventricle. In the famous Framingham Heart Study (see pages 32–33), the thickness of the heart was a better predictor of heart attack and stroke than blood pressure measurements obtained in the doctor's surgery.

With effective treatment of blood pressure, the walls of the heart can actually get thinner. By evaluating the thickness of the heart muscle, as well as the thickness of the inner lining of the carotid artery by doing a carotid ultrasound, I can better distinguish who has white-coat hypertension (blood pressure that seems to be elevated only in the doctor's surgery) from those with truly sustained high blood pressure, which is a threat to their organs.

Follow-up. For patients with high blood pressure and thick heart walls, I repeat the test if there is a significant change in their risk-factor profile or in symptoms related to the heart.

Exercise Stress Test

What is it? The primary purpose of an exercise stress test is to determine your ability to increase bloodflow through your coronary arteries to your heart muscle when your heart is beating faster and/or harder, demanding two to five times the bloodflow it gets at rest.

If you have been feeling symptoms such as chest pain or shortness of breath with exertion, an exercise stress test will help your doctor figure out whether these symptoms are coming from sluggish bloodflow due to a blockage in one or more of your coronary arteries. The stress test will also indicate how severely the blockage is limiting the bloodflow, which is crucial information in deciding whether to recommend an invasive or noninvasive approach to treatment.

Doctors also get other valuable information from a stress test. From watching a patient exercise, we get a good sense of whether the person's symptoms are heart or lung related. For instance, some patients complain of shortness of breath even while they are demonstrating outstanding exercise capacity on the treadmill or bike. And yet they don't appear short of breath to me. These people may have the benign 'sighing' type of shortness of breath I described on page 200. Other patients demonstrate limited exercise capacity with extreme shortness of breath, and yet they still insist they are doing fine. These are the patients I look at much more closely.

Studies from Steven N. Blair, PED, of the Cooper Institute in Dallas, Texas, as well as others, have indicated that overall exercise capacity is an excellent predictor of future health and longevity. The blood pressure response to exercise is a helpful sign of the risk of future complications from hypertension, such as heart attack and stroke.

The two most common types of exercise stress tests are the plain ECG test and the nuclear (or thallium) test. During both tests, you walk on a treadmill or ride a bike, which increases in elevation and/or speed every few minutes. In the plain ECG stress test, leads are applied to your chest, as they are for the basic ECG described on page 203, and tracings are similarly produced. We look for changes on the tracings that indicate compromised bloodflow to the heart muscle.

In the nuclear exercise stress test, two sets of images are taken. The first is taken after a small amount of a radioactive tracer (such as thallium) is injected when you are at rest. This is not a dye, so allergic reactions are not a problem. The second set is done after the tracer is re-injected when you are at peak exercise on the treadmill or bike. The radioactive substance travels to the heart muscle in proportion to the flow of blood. If there is a blockage in one or more of the coronary arteries supplying blood to the bottom of your heart, this area will accumulate less thallium during exercise than other areas with normal bloodflow. The resting and exercise images are then compared and significant blockage will almost always be apparent.

In younger patients in whom I do not suspect heart disease, I use the plain ECG exercise stress test. In older patients, in those with abnormal resting ECGs, and in patients in whom I strongly suspect coronary artery disease, I prefer the nuclear stress test because it gives a better quantification of heart muscle areas with compromised bloodflow.

For patients who cannot exercise, there is a third type of stress test called a *pharmaceutical stress test*. In this test, a drug is injected to dilate the coronary arteries, which allows increased bloodflow unless there is a blockage. Nuclear images are obtained in the same manner described for the nuclear stress test to reflect relative bloodflow during rest and during exercise. A pharmaceutical stress test can also be performed using echocardiography; this is called a *stress echo*. In this, a drug called dobutamine is given intravenously in gradually increasing doses. Dobutamine acts on the heart like adrenaline does, making the heart work harder by pumping harder and faster. An echocardiogram evaluating the pumping function of the heart is performed at rest and during maximal dobutamine stress, and the scans are compared. Regions of heart muscle receiving compromised bloodflow can be identified as areas that do not contract as well during 'stress' as those regions receiving a normal blood supply.

As I explained in Chapter 2, a stress test is a good indicator of the state of a patient's coronary bloodflow at the time of the test. But its ability to predict the future does have limitations. You can accumulate a lot of plaque in your coronary arteries, and even have blockages, yet still maintain normal bloodflow at rest and during exercise. This is because your body may have produced the protective network of collateral blood vessels I described on page 29.

While a stress test is valuable for women as well as men, studies have shown that women have more abnormal exercise ECG stress tests without necessarily having obstructive coronary disease. These women may have a disease of their smaller vessels, which can limit bloodflow and cause chest pain but not necessarily cause a heart attack. Having a nuclear stress test or stress echo rather than a plain ECG stress test helps to reduce the number of false positive tests for women.

Follow-up. If a patient's initial stress test is fine, I normally do not repeat it unless there is a change in the person's symptoms or risk factors. In high-risk patients, including those with known coronary artery disease, I repeat a stress test on a more regular basis.

Carotid Artery Ultrasound

What is it? There are two carotid arteries, which run just under the skin on each side of your neck and supply blood to your brain. Atherosclerosis in the carotid arteries can lead to a stroke. Because the carotids run so close to the surface, they are accessible to ultrasound imaging, which provides exquisite pictures of the vessel walls. In contrast, coronary arteries cannot be well imaged by ultrasound because they run far below the surface of the chest wall, and intervening muscle, bone and lung tissues interfere with the ultrasound signal.

With carotid ultrasound, a water-soluble gel is applied to the skin on your neck to enhance sound wave transmission, then the ultrasound technician moves a transducer over one of your carotid arteries to obtain images. The test, which takes 10 to 15 minutes, provides a measurement of the inner lining of your carotid arteries. This measurement is called the *intimal medial thickness,* and it is a good predictor of heart attack and stroke. Studies show that with risk-factor treatment, you can slow or even reverse the increase in intimal medial thickness. A carotid ultrasound can also image plaque in the carotid arteries as well as bloodflow, revealing any blockages. Like other ultrasound tests, it is quick, safe and painless.

Follow-up. If a patient has cardiac risk factors and an abnormal scan, I follow these abnormalities yearly to help track the effectiveness of the therapy I have prescribed.

STEP

4

GETTING THE RIGHT MEDICATIONS

You're eating a heart-healthy diet and exercising regularly, but your blood pressure and cholesterol numbers – not to mention your triglyceride, C-reactive protein and homocysteine levels – still aren't as good as they should be. Although leading a healthy lifestyle can eliminate or improve most risk factors for heart disease, the later you begin adopting healthy habits, the more likely you are to need the help of medications prescribed by your doctor.

If everyone followed an optimal diet and exercise programme from early childhood on, heart attacks and strokes would be rare. Furthermore, many other chronic diseases of the Western world would also be dramatically reduced. The longer we wait to implement constructive changes in lifestyle, the more likely it is that these measures alone won't be sufficient to undo the damage of too many years of bad eating and sedentary living. This is when the right medications can become lifesaving.

Medications can also make a huge difference in people with a strong genetic predisposition to heart disease. Over the years, I have observed many cases where a patient's optimal lifestyle has delayed but not stopped bad genes from increasing atherosclerosis and causing chest pain or a heart attack. For these people, adding medications to their healthy lifestyle can restack the genetic deck in their favour.

How do you know whether you have reached a stage when a healthy lifestyle isn't enough and you need one or more medications to prevent heart disease? It largely depends on your own risk profile. Once atherosclerosis is present – for example, if you have a high Calcium Score or if you have already experienced a heart attack – then I feel very strongly that medications should be used. I also recommend medications for people who are at moderate risk, but whose risk factors are not responding adequately to lifestyle changes and who are developing atherosclerosis as a result. The decision to take a medication should always be made in consultation with your doctor, but the more you know about your options, the easier it will be for your doctor to counsel you.

Many patients bristle at the suggestion that they take medications, because they think that all medications have side effects. While side effects, as well as effectiveness, have always been a consideration when weighing the pros and cons of drug treatment, there has been real progress in the quality of medications. When I began practising medicine more than 30 years ago, there were relatively few drugs available for treating heart disease, and the ones we could choose from weren't very effective. They often had to be pushed to the limits of their tolerability and be taken several times a day to work. Now we have many more choices. The great majority of heart drugs need to be taken just once daily, and they are more effective and have fewer side effects than their predecessors. Moreover, their benefits and safety have been well documented in many large clinical trials.

Today, more often than not, the benefits of taking medications far outweigh the risks, a point that has not yet registered with many people. Sometimes I find that the usually healthy scepticism of patients regarding taking medications goes too far. When it does, it can interfere with the critical decision to take a potentially lifesaving drug. Or, if a patient does reluctantly decide to take the drug, it can affect their compliance with taking it regularly.

In recent years, the availability of powerful statin drugs for reducing high cholesterol (along with other medications such as prescription niacin and angiotensin-converting enzyme inhibitors) has made the likelihood of having a heart attack or stroke less than ever before, even among high-risk patients. Moreover, thanks to cutting-edge diagnostic tests such as the heart scan and advanced blood testing (which I covered in the previous chapter), we can better identify who would most benefit from drug therapy and be more precise about which drugs to use.

If your doctor has already talked to you about using prescription medications, but you're unsure about whether you should follow the advice, I hope that this chapter will help answer some of your questions. If your doctor hasn't brought up the subject of medications, but you are aware that you may be at risk for a heart attack or stroke, ask your doctor whether medications might reduce that risk. It's possible that you may need more than one drug to achieve the best results. I often combine two or more drugs to get my high-risk patients' bad LDL down to the optimal level of 1.8 mmol/L or below or to treat patients who have multiple risk factors such as high cholesterol, high blood pressure and high triglycerides.

In addition to prescribing medications as needed, I also recommend nutritional supplements – conservatively. Unlike drugs that are regulated, supplements are unregulated and, as a result, can be marketed to the public without undergoing the rigorous scientific review required of drug manufacturers' products. For this and other reasons that I go into on pages 144–45, I much prefer that people get their nutrients from food. However, in rare cases I do recommend supplements that have been scientifically proven to be both safe and effective. For more information on these supplements, see pages 232–38.

Lipid-Lowering Medications

Lipid-lowering medications are designed to reduce levels of bad fats in your blood. They have revolutionized the practice of cardiology and are having a huge impact on the natural history of coronary artery disease. The only problems are that they are not being used often enough and usually not in high enough dosages. On the following pages, I describe some of the drugs that help bring lipids to their ideal levels. Although the primary goal of some of these drugs may be to lower blood fats, they frequently have additional benefits, such as reducing inflammation and helping to prevent the rupture of soft plaque that triggers a heart attack.

Statin Drugs

Before the discovery of statin drugs, I could never have said so unequivocally that the overwhelming majority of heart attacks are preventable. Statins, along with other medications, have changed the prognosis for tens of millions of people who are at risk for heart disease or who already have it.

Statin drugs (or *HMG-CoA reductase inhibitors*) work by inhibiting an enzyme called HMG-CoA, which plays a critical role in the liver's production of cholesterol. If you have high levels of bad LDL cholesterol, you should talk to your doctor about whether taking a statin drug would be helpful. Unfortunately, as I mentioned earlier, only about half of all high-risk people who would benefit from taking statins are actually getting them. By any standard, statins are under-prescribed. I have no doubt that if more people were on statins, there would be far fewer heart attacks and strokes and far less need for angioplasty and bypass surgery.

There are cardiologists, however, who are so enthusiastic about statins that some not so jokingly say that they should be put in the water supply! I don't go quite that far in my endorsement. That's because for low-risk people to take them is costly and exposes them to the possibility of side effects unnecessarily. But for those with multiple risk factors or with established heart disease, statins are a true miracle.

Depending on the dosage and the particular brand, statins have been found to reduce the risk of having a heart attack by 20 to 40 per cent. Moreover, statins can lower bad LDL cholesterol by 20 to 60 per cent. This is their major and most important effect. They can also mildly lower triglycerides and raise good HDL, although they are not used primarily for either of these purposes.

One thing to remember is that statins can't significantly increase the size of small HDL or LDL particles. The first step towards increasing HDL and LDL size is making lifestyle changes. But when modifying your lifestyle doesn't work and more help is needed, niacin (see page 221), and to a lesser degree fibrates (see page 224), can be helpful.

There are several brands of statins and each one is different. They include pravastatin (Lipostat), simvastatin (Zocor), fluvastatin (Lescol), atorvastatin (Lipitor) and rosuvastatin (Crestor). Of the statins, simvastatin and atorvastatin have the strongest evidence that they not only decrease LDL but also prevent heart attacks and the need for invasive procedures.

Recent studies indicate that atorvastatin begins to work to prevent heart attacks earlier than the other statins, possibly due to benefits it has other than just lowering LDL. Pravastatin appears to have the lowest incidence of muscle aches and pains. Fluvastatin used to be the least expensive, but simvastatin is now available as a generic drug and is very reasonably priced. In terms of efficacy in lowering LDL cholesterol at maximum doses, rosuvastatin is first, followed by atorvastatin, simvastatin, pravastatin and finally fluvastatin. (In patients with established heart disease or those who are at significant risk, my goal is to lower LDL to less than 1.8 mmol/L.) In the recent and very encouraging ASTEROID Trial, rosuvastatin was shown to shrink soft atherosclerotic plaque.

Statins appear to have a positive impact on heart disease beyond their effect on cholesterol. Particularly when combined with other drugs or with prescription niacin, statins can cause the regression of soft plaque, which is the primary cause of heart disease. Statins can also reduce inflammation and improve the overall health of the blood vessels.

Some of my patients resist taking statin drugs because they are worried about side effects. While I have never seen a serious liver or kidney problem from any of the statins on the market, I have seen patients who have had heart attacks after refusing to take a statin because of their fear of complications. I want to stress that the chance of sustaining liver damage from taking a statin is exceedingly small and that I have never seen a case of it in my practice. While liver enzymes may become elevated, discontinuing the statin brings them back to normal (you might also try another statin as an alternative). Less serious side effects, such as muscle cramps, particularly in the toes at night, as well as general muscle pains are fairly common in my experience. These muscle pains may be due to the fact that statin drugs may deplete muscle cells of coenzyme Q10 (CoQ10), an anti-oxidant produced by the body that is involved in energy production. I have found that taking supplemental CoQ10, which is sold over-the-counter at many pharmacies and health-food shops, can sometimes help relieve these pains.

The most serious complication of statins is an inflammation and breakdown of muscle fibre called *rhabdomyolysis*. This is extremely rare in otherwise healthy patients, and I have never seen a case using the currently available statins. This complication is heralded by severe muscle weakness and soreness that feels similar to awakening with flu so severe you can hardly get out of bed. This problem is completely reversible with prompt attention. So if you are on a statin and have any concern, stop the medication and consult your doctor. The treatment of cholesterol requires medication for months and years. A few days or weeks off the medication is inconsequential.

HOLD THE GRAPEFRUIT JUICE

If you're taking a statin or a blood pressure drug, you should ask your doctor about whether it is safe for you to drink grapefruit juice. Grapefruit contains natural chemicals that inhibit the enzyme CYP3A4, which is involved in the metabolism of about half of all prescription drugs. As a result, drinking grapefruit juice could increase the potency of a medication, and drinking a lot of it can potentially cause side effects. For example, mixing grapefruit juice with some statins increases the risk of muscle toxicity. No need to worry about grapefruit juice if you're not on a statin, or about other citrus juices, because they don't contain the same enzyme-blocking chemical as grapefruit juice.

Niacin

Also called *nicotinic acid*, niacin is a B vitamin (vitamin B$_3$) that you can buy over-the-counter, but I recommend taking it in prescription form because of the pharmaceutical industry's quality assurance. Niacin is a potent elevator of HDL, particularly the large HDL particles that are associated with the greatest protection from progressive atherosclerosis. Both alone and in combination with a statin, niacin has been shown to slow or reverse atherosclerosis and prevent recurrent heart attacks and strokes.

Prescription niacin is available in an slow-release form called Niaspan, which has undergone rigorous scientific testing. In fact, it's one of the few vitamin-based therapies that is approved by the US Food and Drug Administration. Since the supplement industry is largely unregulated, I feel more confident prescribing a product that is guaranteed to contain what the label says it does. While good brands of nonprescription niacin are available, some brands lack potency or have even been found to be dangerous. So if you choose an over-the-counter form, please do it in consultation with your doctor. It is also important that your doctor monitors your response to niacin, including doing periodic liver function tests.

Here are some of the ways that niacin can improve your blood lipids:

- It is one of the few treatments proven to raise HDL ('good') cholesterol, and it can raise it by 15 to 24 per cent.

- It not only reduces bad LDL cholesterol by 5 to 25 per cent, it enlarges the small, dense LDL particles that move into your artery walls so easily.

- It can change small HDL cholesterol particles into the large variety that can remove more cholesterol from vessel walls.

- It can lower triglyceride levels by 20 to 50 per cent. As I have explained, triglycerides are a blood fat that is associated with prediabetes and related to small LDL, small HDL and low total HDL levels.

- It is the only medication that effectively lowers the level of lipoprotein (a), which is unaffected by diet or exercise.

It is not enough for doctors to recommend a medication that has favourable effects on blood lipids unless we can also show that it has the predicted clinical effects, such as slowing atherosclerosis and preventing heart attacks. Niacin passes this test with flying colours, as Dr B. Greg Brown's HDL-Atherosclerosis Treatment Study (known as the HATS trial) showed. The study, published in 2001, involved 160 patients with atherosclerosis who had low HDL levels, on average 0.8 mmol/L. (Anything under 1.0 mmol/L is considered a risk factor for heart attack.) The study combined niacin plus a statin drug, simvastatin (Zocor). Earlier studies had already shown that statin drugs alone could reduce the risk of heart attack by 20 to 40 per cent. But those taking niacin plus the statin drug regime reduced the number of heart attacks and strokes by an astonishing 90 per cent when compared to those taking a placebo (dummy pill)!

The results of the HATS trial were so good that the US National Institutes of Health recently launched a larger trial involving more than 3000 patients. This trial, which has been named AIM HIGH: Niacin Plus Statin to Prevent Vascular Events, will follow patients for 5 years, with results due in 2010.

Yet another study, called the ARBITER-2 trial, published in the journal *Circulation* in 2004, evaluated the potential of niacin to slow atherosclerosis in the carotid arteries leading to the brain. The study involved 167 heart patients. Some added high-dose niacin therapy to a statin drug regime. Others took a statin drug alone. Carotid ultrasound was performed to measure the thickness of the lining of the carotid arteries in both groups of patients. As I explained on page 214, the thicker the lining of the carotid arteries, the greater the degree of atherosclerosis and the higher the risk of heart attack and stroke. Patients taking the statin plus niacin showed a carotid thickness that was 68 per cent less than that of the statin-only group, suggesting that niacin had slowed the progression of the atherosclerosis. Niacin also appeared to be particularly effective at slowing the rate of thickening in those patients with insulin resistance. What's even more remarkable is that the niacin-enhanced group had an increase in HDL cholesterol of 21 per cent. Given the difficulty of raising HDL, this increase is very significant. Niacin appears to be a perfect partner for the statins because its strongest effects are on the blood lipids that are least affected by statins.

So if niacin is so good, why aren't more people who are at risk for heart disease taking it? The reason is that niacin is more difficult to take than statins because of its side effects. In particular, several hours after it is taken, niacin commonly causes a 'flushing' reaction that lasts about 45 minutes and may also be associated with itching. This side effect, which is not toxic, occurs because niacin dilates small blood vessels supplying the skin. The flushing reaction can be limited when niacin is taken with food and an aspirin, and it usually disappears with continued use. But when patients are not warned that flushing might occur and assured that it's not an allergic reaction, they often become alarmed and stop taking niacin. When I tell them what might occur in advance, I find that most patients don't overreact to flushing and end up tolerating niacin well.

Other, less common side effects that can occur with niacin include rashes, abdominal pain and elevated liver enzymes. And some over-the-counter niacin products in the past have been associated with more serious liver problems (which have not been a significant problem with prescription niacin). Niacin may also increase blood sugar slightly, but this rarely becomes a problem. Overall, I have found niacin to be a safe and effective medication, but whether you take it in prescription or over-the-counter form, you absolutely must be monitored by your doctor.

Ezetimibe (Ezetrol)

Ezetimibe is a new class of lipid-lowering drug that acts by blocking the absorption of cholesterol in the small intestine. Marketed under the brand name Ezetrol, it can be used alone (by those who can't tolerate statins) or in combination with statins to manage high cholesterol.

Ezetimibe is useful for patients who cannot get their LDL cholesterol low enough by taking statins alone or who are not good candidates for niacin because of its side effects. When combined with a statin, ezetimibe dramatically lowers LDL cholesterol, and it does this almost invariably without adding side effects. In patients who have trouble taking anything more than the lowest dose of a statin, the addition of ezetimibe often allows them to achieve the goal of an LDL cholesterol of less than 1.8 mmol/L.

In addition to helping to lower LDL, ezetimibe can also lower levels of C-reactive protein (CRP), a marker for inflammation. As I discussed previously, high levels of CRP are an important risk factor for heart attack and stroke. One study found that when combined with a statin drug, ezetimibe has twice the CRP-lowering power of a statin drug alone.

The good news about ezetimibe is that it is easy to tolerate and you only need to take it once a day. The only serious side effect is a rare allergic reaction associated with a rash.

Fibrates

Fibrates are a class of drugs that have been prescribed since before the statin era, which began in 1987. The first fibrate, clofibrate, was withdrawn from the market after many years of use because of adverse side effects. However, there are currently four fibrates on the market in the UK, gemfibrozil (Lopid), fenofibrate (Lipantil), ciprofibrate (Modalin) and bezafibrate (Bezalip), that are well tolerated and quite safe. Gemfibrozil has been around the longest and is taken twice a day. Because it's available as a generic, it is quite affordable. The newest fibrate is fenofibrate, which is taken once daily and is generally safe when used in combination with statins, an important attribute.

The fibrates are most effective at reducing triglycerides. They also increase HDL and the size of HDL and LDL particles, though they do not perform this function as effectively as niacin. Like niacin, their strengths are in areas where statins are weak, making the statin-fibrate combination attractive.

What about fibrates' track record in clinical trials showing an actual decrease in heart attacks? While not as extensive as the evidence for statins, recent studies suggest that fibrates can reduce the risk of death from cardiovascular disease. This is especially true in patients with lipid problems due to prediabetes and diabetes. An 18-year follow-up to the Helsinki Heart Study published in 2006 in the *Archives of Internal Medicine* showed that heart patients with a high body mass index (BMI) and a high triglyceride level (two risk factors for prediabetes) who were taking gemfibrozil had a 71 per cent reduction in death from coronary artery disease and a 33 per cent reduction in death from all causes. Very impressive.

While usually very well tolerated, fibrates occasionally cause stomach upset and rarely cause muscle weakness. Your liver function should be monitored by your doctor.

Bile Acid Sequestrants

Also known as *resins*, bile acid sequestrants were among the earliest cholesterol-lowering medications to be developed. They were used in the landmark Lipid Research Clinics Coronary Primary Prevention Trial (LRC-CPPT), a 10-year study completed in 1983, which was the first study to demonstrate that lowering cholesterol resulted in a statistically significant decrease in heart disease. While the trial actually showed a very small decrease in heart attack rates, bile acid sequestrants were the best drugs available for lowering cholesterol back then, even though they were and are difficult to take. Luckily, we've come a long way since the LRC-CPPT.

Bile acid sequestrants work by binding with cholesterol-containing bile acids in the intestines and removing them in the stool, thus preventing their absorption into the bloodstream. Like ezetimibe, they work exclusively in the intestine, but unlike ezetimibe, they have to be taken several times a day and are much more likely to cause abdominal problems, mainly pain and bloating. They are currently sold under the brand names Questran (cholestyramine), Colestid (colestipol) and WelChol (colesevelam).

Bile acid sequestrants on their own can lower LDL cholesterol by up to 20 per cent and by up to 40 per cent when used in combination with statins and/or prescription niacin for potentially better results. However, since these medications can actually raise triglyceride levels, they are not appropriate for people with elevated or borderline high triglycerides.

In my practice, I rarely prescribe bile acid sequestrants because my patients find them difficult to take. In powder form, they have to be mixed with water or juice, and some people have trouble getting the mixture down. Even when taken in tablet form, bile acid sequestrants still have to be washed down with lots of water. In any form, these drugs can cause troublesome gastrointestinal symptoms, notably constipation, bloating, nausea and wind. Moreover, if not taken at the proper time, they can interfere with the absorption of other medications, such as beta-blockers, blood thinners and thiazide diuretics.

I mention bile acid sequestrants here because they can be useful for high-risk people who can't take statins but need to get their LDL down to the lowest level possible.

Blood Pressure Medications

Today we have some wonderful medications that help control blood pressure. That hasn't always been the case. When I first began practising medicine, diuretics (water pills) were the most commonly prescribed drugs for high blood pressure. Diuretics in low dosages relax arterial walls and thus lower blood pressure. In high dosages, they further lower blood pressure by decreasing your blood volume. With less fluid to pump, the heart doesn't have to work as hard and blood pressure falls.

Although diuretics can reduce blood pressure, there are several problems with them. In order to be effective as a sole therapy, diuretics have to be taken in fairly high doses, causing not only the loss of excess water, but also the loss of significant amounts of the mineral potassium. And this can be life-threatening.

Because we now have so many other blood pressure–lowering medications, doctors have the luxury of using diuretics at much lower dosages; these are not only very safe but also very effective. Often, in patients whose blood pressure is resistant to other medications, adding a very low dose of a diuretic can make a big difference. In addition, there are many combination medications available that combine a low dosage of a diuretic with another blood pressure medication, such as an angiotensin-converting enzyme inhibitor or beta-blocker. This allows for the convenience of once-a-day dosing in just one pill. Diuretics have also stood the test of time, whereas most of the other blood pressure medications I used during my early training have become obsolete.

The blood pressure medications covered below have been part of a true revolution in the treatment of high blood pressure and the prevention of heart attacks and strokes. No longer do patients have to deal with medications for blood pressure that need to be taken many times a day or commonly have side effects.

Angiotensin-Converting Enzyme Inhibitors and Angiotensin II Receptor Blockers

Angiotensin-converting enzyme (ACE) inhibitors and angiotensin II receptor blockers (ARBs) are two related classes of blood pressure medications that are safe, well tolerated and have positive effects beyond blood pressure lowering.

Introduced years before the ARBs, ACE inhibitors relax (dilate) blood vessels by blocking the formation of angiotensin II, a substance that constricts blood vessels and is itself a risk factor for heart attacks. In the large Heart Outcomes Prevention Evaluation (HOPE) trial conducted at 267 medical centres around the world from 1996 to 1999, the ACE inhibitor ramipril (Altace) was found to prevent both heart attacks and strokes beyond its ability to lower blood pressure. We think we know why. ACE inhibitors actually improve the health of the endothelium, the lining of the arterial wall. The HOPE study also found that fewer patients taking Altace went on to develop diabetes compared to those taking a placebo (dummy pill).

ACE inhibitors are also standard therapy for patients with heart failure who do not have high blood pressure. When on an ACE inhibitor, these patients have fewer heart attacks as well as fewer episodes of heart failure. Because of their apparent benefits for preventing heart attacks, I use ACE inhibitors in high-risk patients with blood pressures in the high-normal range.

Most people can tolerate ACE inhibitors well, but a common side effect is a dry cough. This cough is not dangerous and does not indicate a lung problem. It is the result of an increase in histamine in the bloodstream. Histamine is a chemical that can cause the dilation of small blood vessels, but in excess, it can cause allergic symptoms. Due to its effect on blood vessels, the increased histamine may in fact be part of the way ACE inhibitors work. Therefore, I only discontinue the ACE inhibitor if the patient – or his or her spouse – finds the cough bothersome. A far rarer but important adverse reaction to ACE inhibitors is angioedema, a type of allergic reaction that causes swelling (*oedema*) of the extremities, and notably the tongue, and requires prompt medical attention.

Among the ACE inhibitors commonly prescribed are benazepril (Lotensin), captopril (Capoten), enalapril (Vasotec), ramipril (Altace), lisinopril (Zestril), trandolapril (Gopten) and perindopril (Coversyl). Most of these are now available in generic form.

ARBs are closely related to ACE inhibitors but are almost never associated with cough. Like ACE inhibitors, they are generally once-daily medications and are very well tolerated. There are now so many ARBs available that it is hard to keep up with the minor differences between them. But while there may be small differences between ARBs, they all appear to be safe, effective and an excellent alternative to ACE inhibitors. In addition to lowering blood pressure, ARBs may help prevent people with prediabetes from getting full-blown diabetes and those who already have diabetes from getting kidney disease.

Some patients may benefit from taking a combination of an ARB and an ACE inhibitor. And ACE inhibitors and ARBs are also available in convenient dosages combined with a low-dose diuretic (hydrochlorothiazide). Among the most commonly prescribed ARBs are losartan hydrochloride (Cozaar), telmisartan (Micardis), valsartan (Diovan), olmesartan (Olmetec), candesartan (Atacand), eprosartan (Teveten) and irbesartan (Avapro).

Beta-Blockers

Beta-blockers are a class of drugs that work by blocking the action of the hormone epinephrine (also called *adrenaline*). This 'fight or flight' hormone is what causes the many changes we associate with stress, including a rapid heart rate, increased blood pressure, perspiration, tremor and anxiety. Adrenaline also enhances the ability of your blood to clot and helps promote constriction of the arteries, both crucial in the face of an acute traumatic injury.

The first beta-blocker, which became available in the 1970s, was propranolol (Inderal). I used it during my cardiology training for patients with chest pain on exertion because it blunts the increase in heart rate and demand for blood during exercise that causes angina (chest pain). Propranolol was also commonly used to treat high blood pressure. Back then, propranolol had to be taken several times a day and in much higher dosages than we use today because of the absence of other medications for angina and high blood pressure. Today, I still prescribe it, but in lower dosages, and I use many of the other beta-blockers that are now available as once-daily medications.

If you've already had a heart attack, taking a beta-blocker can help reduce the risk of having another. In fact, national recommendations advise that heart attack patients be given a prescription for a beta-blocker upon discharge from the hospital. Because beta-blockers decrease the strength of the heart's contractions, they were always studiously avoided in patients with heart failure due to weak or damaged heart muscle. But in the 1990s, studies demonstrated that beta-blockers actually improve the outcome of patients with a history of heart failure, and they are now standard treatment for patients with weak heart muscle.

The main limitations in taking beta-blockers are fatigue, weakness and a slow heart rate, which are primarily associated with moderate to high dosages. I have often seen older patients (and less often younger ones) who are taking a beta-blocker complain of a lack of energy, but when I reduce their dosage, a dramatic improvement results. Beta-blockers may also cause depression in some patients; if this happens, I lower the dosage or substitute another medication.

Patients taking beta-blockers must have their heart rate monitored regularly, since occasionally the heart rate can slow enough to cause symptoms. Beta-blockers may also have an adverse effect on lipids, in particular a lowering of good HDL. A relatively new beta-blocker, carvedilol (Coreg), is an exception. Not only does it have no adverse effect on lipids, it improves a patient's sensitivity to insulin, thereby having a favourable effect on patients with diabetes or prediabetes.

Currently many beta-blockers are available, and several are in generic formulations. Beta-blockers have also become more convenient to take, with once-a-day or twice-a-day dosing. Besides propranolol and carvedilol, beta-blockers that are often prescribed include atenolol, bisoprolol and metoprolol.

Calcium Channel Blockers

Calcium channel blockers (also called *calcium antagonists*) dilate arteries, which improves bloodflow and reduces blood pressure. They are also used to treat angina (chest pain), and some forms are prescribed to treat abnormal heart rhythms (arrhythmias). Don't be confused by the word *calcium* in *calcium channel blockers*; it refers to their mode of action, but they have no effect on calcium levels in the blood.

Calcium channel blockers are well-tolerated, once-a-day medications that may be used effectively in combination with many of the other blood pressure medications discussed here. Their effect on preventing heart attacks is not as well documented as it is for other classes of blood pressure medications, but some studies indicate that some calcium channel blocker formulations might retard the progression of atherosclerosis.

The most common complaint I see with calcium channel blockers is ankle swelling. This is due to their ability to dilate veins in the legs, allowing fluid to settle there. The swelling is not a sign of other problems and is really only an adverse cosmetic effect. It should not be treated with regular doses of diuretics. If the swelling is excessive, then discontinuing the calcium channel blocker or trying another one is necessary.

Among the calcium channel blockers commonly used are diltiazem, nifedipine, verapamil, felodipine and amlodipine.

Aspirin

Your grandmother used to take aspirin for all her aches and pains, but this old-time remedy is now considered routine *preventive* medicine. As well known and inexpensive as aspirin is, I find that it is often hard for patients to take its heart attack–preventing effects seriously. Dr Charles Hennekens, who headed the famous 1980 Physicians' Health Study at Harvard, which clearly established low-dose aspirin as a life-saving drug, often remarks that if aspirin were much more expensive and had many more side effects, it might be taken more seriously.

Aspirin is both an anti-inflammatory and an inhibitor of blood clotting (it reduces the stickiness of blood platelets and prevents them from clumping together). This means that if you do rupture a plaque, injure the vessel wall, and induce blood clot formation, aspirin will help prevent the clot from growing to a size that limits bloodflow and causes an acute coronary syndrome. Aspirin can decrease your chance of experiencing a heart attack by about 25 per cent, which is pretty impressive. For this reason, I consider it a major weapon in the fight against heart disease.

The American Heart Association has long recommended low-dose aspirin for people who already have had a heart attack, unstable angina, or a stroke caused by a blood clot (*ischaemic stroke*). They also recommend it for people who have had transient ischaemic attacks, or TIAs. Transient ischaemic attacks are interruptions in bloodflow to the brain, similar to those of a stroke, but they resolve completely over a period of minutes without permanent effects. They can be precursors of a stroke, however.

Since the Physicians' Health Study found that men who took 325 milligrams of aspirin every other day reduced their risk of a first heart attack by 44 per cent, doctors have been quite positive about prescribing aspirin to male patients. But for years we didn't know whether aspirin would help women. As it turns out, there does appear to be a difference in the way aspirin affects men and women. A major 2005 study published in the *New England Journal of Medicine* involving 39,876 initially healthy women found that women over the age of 65 who took 100 milligrams of aspirin every other day experienced a 26 per cent decline in the risk of having either a heart attack or stroke. Unlike its effect on men, in this study, aspirin did not offer women under the age of 65 a risk reduction in heart attack, but it did reduce the risk of stroke by 17 per cent for the total study population.

There are a few caveats that go along with taking aspirin. Don't start popping aspirin on your own without first consulting your doctor. Aspirin can cause stomach bleeding, and it should not be used by people who have or are prone to gastrointestinal ulcers. If you take aspirin regularly, you should avoid alcohol, which can also irritate the stomach lining. Because aspirin is a nonsteroidal anti-inflammatory drug (NSAID), it should not be taken with other NSAIDs, such as ibuprofen (Nurofen) or naproxen (Naprosyn). And because it can thin the blood, avoid taking it with anticlotting medications such as warfarin.

I suspect that you have read advice that tells you to take an aspirin if you think that you are having a heart attack in order to dissolve the clot. You should indeed take a full-strength, preferably uncoated, adult aspirin (325 milligrams) if you think you are having a heart attack. If you think that you are having a stroke, however, *don't take aspirin*. Some strokes are caused by a bleed in the brain. Taking aspirin may only increase the bleeding. (For information on the symptoms of heart attack and stroke, see pages 239–46.)

Dietary Supplements

When I tell patients that they need to take one or more medications to improve their cholesterol profile, many of them ask me whether a natural, over-the-counter dietary supplement would do the job just as well. The answer is 'No'. As I mentioned earlier, because the supplement industry is not regulated, most supplements have never undergone the rigorous scientific testing that is required for approval of a pharmaceutical product. Moreover, the research that has been performed on specific supplements – notably, antioxidants – has been very disappointing.

One of these antioxidants, vitamin E, which has long been taken by people to help protect against heart disease, was in the news not long ago. Although I don't recommend vitamin E to my patients, I was still surprised when I read that a review of 19 published vitamin E studies had found that taking a daily dose of 400 IU or more of vitamin E may *increase* mortality from all causes. People who took such a dose of vitamin E were found to be 10 per cent more likely to die a premature death than those who were given a placebo (dummy pill). According to the report, 'High-dosage vitamin E supplements may increase all-cause mortality and should be avoided.' I did, and do, recommend that my patients get their vitamin E from foods.

If people were surprised by the vitamin E study, they were shocked by the results of an even more recent study of B vitamins. The conventional wisdom has been to take folic acid, B_{12} and B_6 to decrease an elevated homocysteine level. But the 2005 Norwegian Vitamin Trial made us all reassess our position when it comes to treating elevated homocysteine with B vitamins. In this study, some heart attack survivors took 40 milligrams of vitamin B_6, 400 micrograms of B_{12} and 800 micrograms of folic acid for nearly 3½ years. The vitamins did, in fact, lower these subjects' homocysteine levels. But, to everyone's surprise, these vitamin-takers had a 20 per cent increased risk of having another heart attack or a stroke compared with people who took a placebo.

As far as the antioxidant vitamins in general are concerned, we all thought they would be helpful weapons against heart disease because of what we had gleaned from some basic laboratory studies. However, three very large clinical trials, the HOPE trial, the GISSI heart study and the Heart Protection Study, failed to document any benefits from antioxidant vitamins. The good news is that neither did they document any adverse effects. These studies tested antioxidant cocktails in fighting heart disease as well as nonvascular disease. The results showed that antioxidants did not prevent heart disease, cancer or any other class of disease.

We are just beginning to figure out why the antioxidant vitamins haven't fulfilled their promise. Relatively recent research has shown that fruits and vegetables contain literally thousands of micronutrients (see page 146) that interact in ways we don't yet understand. The well-known antioxidant vitamins – A, C and E – are just three small contributors to this huge quantity and variety of potentially healthy nutrients in our natural, unprocessed foods. Until we learn a lot more about isolating the most important nutrients and putting them in pill form, our best strategy is to consume a wide variety of fruits and vegetables. This is what the hunter-gatherers did, and we have not been as healthy since.

Besides the absence of clinical evidence supporting supplements, I have another concern about them. What you see on the label is not always what you get because, as I noted earlier, the manufacturers are not required to meet the same rigorous production and quality standards that manufacturers of prescription drugs are.

A number of investigations have shown that some supplements contain only small amounts of the advertised ingredients or offer the ingredients in a form that is not effective. If you want to use supplements, how do you protect yourself against fraud? One option is to purchase pharmaceutical-grade products that must meet stringent standards. Many doctors and other health-care professionals sell such high-grade supplements (I don't), as do some online pharmacies. If you don't want to go this route, at least purchase products produced by major, well-known manufacturers.

A handful of supplements have withstood extensive scientific review, however, and I actually do use them in my practice.

Omega-3 Fatty Acid Supplements (Fish Oils)

At the present time, few supplements have been established as being safe and effective additions to cardiology care. One that has and that stands out as a valuable addition to a healthy lifestyle is omega-3 fatty acids, also known as *fish oil*. The active ingredients in omega-3s are docosahexaenoic acid (DHA) and eicosapentaenoic acid (EPA), and both are listed on the label. A total of between 1000 and 2000 milligrams of fish oil a day is recommended. If you eat a lot of cold-water oily fish, such as salmon, herring and sardines, however, a supplement may not be necessary.

Omega-3s are a safe and effective way to lower significantly elevated triglycerides, but they must be taken at a much higher dose than that suggested above. Recently a prescription omega-3 was introduced under the name Omacor. Because it has a high level of quality assurance, I now prescribe it for my patients with high triglycerides.

In 2002, the American Heart Association recommended DHA and EPA for patients who have coronary artery disease as long as they obtain their doctor's approval. According to a Scientific Statement published by the American Heart Association in its journal *Circulation,* members of the association's Nutrition Committee concluded that 'omega-3 fatty acids have been shown in epidemiological and clinical trials to reduce the incidence of cardiovascular disease'. The statement also noted that a daily intake of 0.5 to 1.8 grams of EPA plus DHA through supplements or eating oily fish significantly reduced mortality among people who had already had a heart attack.

How does fish oil help prevent heart disease? It does so by lowering triglycerides and reducing inflammation. It also reduces the risk of abnormal heart rhythms, including those that can cause sudden death. Moreover, fish oil does its good work without significantly affecting either LDL or HDL.

In addition to being heart-protective, omega-3s have also been found to be helpful to most of our other organs, including the brain, lungs, bowels and skin. Omega-3s may also help prevent Alzheimer's disease. This is a supplement I take myself and that I strongly recommend.

Does it matter which brand of fish oil you take? According to a July 2003 survey conducted by *Consumer Reports,* all of the top 16 brands of fish oil have the same high quality and purity and contain the amounts of EPA and DHA described on the label. For this reason, the organization recommends that you shop by price.

Fish oil does occasionally have one minor side effect – 'fishy burps' and a fishy taste in the mouth that some patients do not like. In recent years, however, enteric-coated capsules and tablets that minimize these effects have appeared on the market. The coating delays absorption until the supplements reach the small intestine. (Refrigerating your fish oil capsules will also help prevent that fishy taste.) As a cautionary note, fish oil can increase bleeding time, so anyone taking blood thinners or who has plans for elective surgery should tell their doctor that they are taking a fish oil supplement.

Another reason to consider a fish oil supplement is concern over the presence of mercury and other pollutants in fish. While we all need to be careful, pregnant and nursing women need to be especially vigilant. There's also the likelihood that farm-fed fish may not have the same omega-3 levels as wild fish. If you take a good fish oil supplement, you don't have to worry about mercury or getting lower than expected levels of omega-3s.

Plant Sterols and Stanols (Phytosterols)

Other natural substances with proven efficacy are stanol esters and sterol esters. These plant extracts (known collectively as *phytosterols*) have been shown to help lower LDL cholesterol. They are sold as dietary supplements in softgel form in health-food shops and are added to foods such as margarine, snack bars and salad dressings.

THINK BEFORE YOU SWALLOW

Be sure to tell your doctor about all the medications and nutritional supplements you take regularly, whether they're prescription or over-the-counter. When taken in combination with other drugs, many otherwise safe medications can interact with each other, causing potentially dangerous side effects. This is also true for supplements. Some supplements can increase the effect of prescription drugs, or of each other, which could also increase the risk for side effects. It's best to err on the side of caution and check with your doctor about possible drug and supplement interactions.

Plant sterol esters and plant stanol esters are structurally similar to cholesterol, and because of this, they block cholesterol absorption in your small intestine. In this way, the esters act like the medications we described on the previous pages that decrease cholesterol absorption and thereby lower cholesterol levels in your blood. They are very safe and have no apparent side effects.

In fact, plant sterols and stanols were included among the Therapeutic Lifestyle Changes recommended by the US National Cholesterol Education Program panel of experts in 2002. And a 2005 study published in the *American Journal of Cardiology* also found them valuable. It concluded that 'recommended intakes of about 2 to 2.5 grams a day of products enriched with plant stanol/sterol esters lower plasma LDL cholesterol levels by 10 to 14 per cent without any reported side effects. Thus, plant stanols/sterols can be considered to be effective and safe cholesterol-lowering functional food ingredients.' They were also recommended by the Joint British Societies in their 2005 document on 'Prevention of Cardiovascular Disease in Clinical Practice'.

If you have slightly elevated LDL, taking sterol/stanol supplements and eating products fortified with plant sterol/stanol esters as part of an otherwise healthy diet could be enough to bring your LDL down to optimal levels. If you are already taking medications to lower your LDL cholesterol, sterols and stanols may bring it down even further.

Fibre Supplements

As I noted earlier, Western societies consume only a fraction of the amount of fibre that is considered ideal. This is unfortunate because fibre from food or supplements can help to lower your cholesterol. It also helps to slow digestion, which can prevent surges in blood sugar. For this reason, fibre can be very important for those with prediabetes or diabetes who need to control their blood sugar. It is also essential for good bowel function. If you adopt the South Beach Diet, as I recommend in Step 1 of my heart programme, you will get plenty of fibre from eating whole grains, whole fruits and vegetables. But if you are on the go or are concerned that you are not regularly getting enough fibre from your diet, fibre supplements such as psyllium, methylcellulose and polycarbophil are safe and effective. Just be sure to take them with plenty of water.

· · · · · · ·

Bottom line: Medicines and supplements are not magic bullets. They are simply one part of the South Beach Heart Programme. And while they are invaluable components of my prevention strategy, they are not – and shouldn't be – substitutes for a healthy lifestyle. I can't say this too many times: the earlier you adopt a healthy way of life, the less likely you are to need medications to prevent a heart attack or stroke.

ARE YOU HAVING A HEART ATTACK OR STROKE?

As a preventive cardiologist, I don't see many heart attacks or strokes in my practice, yet I feel that it is extremely important that my patients be aware of the symptoms of each.

You might assume that you'd know if you were having a heart attack or stroke, but the fact is, many people don't. One problem is denial. Even when symptoms of a heart attack are classic – chest pain and tightness in the chest – it is often our instinct to deny the worst and assume we are having indigestion. As I described in Chapter 8, this can even happen to a doctor, with fatal consequences. On the other hand, the symptoms for both heart attack and stroke can be subtle and confusing. And while you're trying to figure out what's wrong, you might be wasting precious time. If you think for even a moment that you're having a heart attack or stroke, remember, every minute counts. The earlier you get treatment, the better your chances of survival. We have great tools for interrupting a heart attack as it's occurring, but they can only be applied in patients who seek medical attention in time.

I urge you to read this section. Learn the symptoms. More importantly, be prepared to act. Have an emergency plan in place ahead of time in the event that you or someone you love has a heart attack or stroke. In addition, consider learning cardiopulmonary resuscitation (CPR) at a St John Ambulance or Red Cross centre near you (see Helpful Resources, page 247). Or, if you already have learned it, take a refresher course. As far as a home defibrillator is concerned, it certainly can be lifesaving if it is kept available and ready for immediate use in case of emergency.

Is It a Heart Attack?

Not all heart attacks conform to the stereotype of a man clutching his chest in pain. And nearly half the time, it's not a man whose heart is under assault – it's a woman. And women often experience heart attacks a bit differently than men.

Here are some important symptoms:

- Chest pain is common for both sexes. It could feel like heaviness, burning or squeezing in the centre of the chest. Some people describe the discomfort in terms of tightness or pressure, which may radiate from the chest to either arm, the jaw, neck or back.

- Less common symptoms for both sexes include breaking out in a cold sweat, general weakness, nausea, shortness of breath, dizziness and/or lightheadedness and/or discomfort or pain between the shoulder blades.

- *Women are more likely than men* to complain of the less common symptoms listed above, as well as jaw and back pain, unusual fatigue and trouble sleeping due to the pain. They may also have a sense that something is terribly wrong or feel an impending sense of doom. Because these are not necessarily the typical symptoms, and women still often perceive themselves as being less likely to experience a heart attack than men, they are slower to seek medical attention and therefore are at greater risk of dying from a heart attack than men.

Brief episodes of chest pain or breathlessness and/or discomfort or pain between the shoulder blades may occur weeks before a heart attack, especially upon exertion. You may first notice symptoms while exercising or walking up a flight of steps, or even during sex, if that's the most demanding physical activity you engage in. These symptoms could be angina, brief periods when the bloodflow is temporarily cut off from a portion of the heart.

If you have any of the symptoms described on the opposite page, especially if you've never experienced them before, and even if they come and go, call 999 for an ambulance and then take one 325-milligram, preferably uncoated, aspirin. An aspirin can help break up the blood clot that is causing the heart attack. (If you are allergic to aspirin or think you're having a stroke, don't take it.)

How do you know whether it's indigestion, angina or a heart attack? Many people get chest pains, the great majority of which do not signal the presence of a heart problem. My standard advice is, if you have a symptom that is new and does not represent an established pattern, call 999 immediately for an ambulance. The modern, well-equipped ambulance is a bit like Accident and Emergency (A&E) brought to your doorstep, and the paramedic team can perform CPR or use a defibrillator to restore normal heart rhythm if need be. Calling 999 is certainly safer than taking yourself to the hospital (if you must, ask someone else to drive you or go with you).

When you arrive in A&E, immediately communicate your concern that you are having a heart attack and describe your symptoms. This is not the time to be shy about asserting yourself. At the hospital, you will be given an electrocardiogram (ECG), a noninvasive test used to check for any sign of injury to the heart muscle and to detect an irregular heartbeat. If, based on the ECG and your symptoms, the doctor judges that you are having an acute coronary syndrome (a heart attack or unstable angina), he or she will treat you immediately. If the ECG is inconclusive, a blood test that identifies certain heart enzymes will confirm whether or not you are having a heart attack. These enzymes are substances that perform vital functions in the heart muscle; they leak out of dying cells into the bloodstream during a heart attack.

If you are having a heart attack, you will most likely be sent for an invasive angiogram or given a clot-busting drug intravenously. There are also times when these approaches may not be appropriate and medical therapy may be the best treatment. Do whatever your doctor tells you to do. Now is not the time to talk about aggressive prevention, demand a noninvasive heart scan, or get a second opinion. Now is the time for *aggressive intervention*. In the event of a heart attack, angioplasty, bypass surgery and clot busters can be true lifesavers.

Women, take note: Many studies indicate that women are more likely to sustain a heart attack without the classic symptoms, such as chest pain, described on the preceding pages. This raises the possibility of misdiagnosis by both the patient and the doctor. Women may only experience the less typical symptoms, such as shortness of breath, weakness or dizziness. As a woman, you have to be extra vigilant to make sure that an ECG and heart enzyme test are performed if you are experiencing symptoms that are new and that concern you.

As I said in Chapter 3, whether you're a man or woman, once you've had a heart attack, you have a 20 per cent chance of dying within 10 years of the first attack, unless you have significantly altered the risk factors that caused the heart attack in the first place. That's why, as soon as you begin recovering from a first heart attack, it's time to begin an aggressive prevention programme to make sure that it never happens again.

Heart attack victims, take note: According to a Mayo Clinic study, for the first month after having a heart attack, your risk of having a stroke is 44 times higher than normal. The risk for stroke declines rapidly after the first month; nevertheless, anyone who has just had a heart attack should be familiar with the symptoms of stroke (see page 245).

When Chest Pain Isn't a Heart Attack

Almost all of us will experience chest pain from time to time. In my experience, the most common cause of chest pain is reflux of stomach acid into the oesophagus, widely known as GERD (gastroesophageal reflux disease). If the oesophagus goes into spasm, it can cause severe chest pain that closely mimics the symptoms of a heart attack. Muscle spasm can also cause chest pain, and women may experience chest discomfort under the left breast due to muscle strain. Transient sharp pains or 'sticks in the chest' lasting for only seconds are frequent complaints that are also uncharacteristic of limited coronary bloodflow. However, if you experience any chest discomfort, especially if you have risk factors for heart disease, do not self-diagnose. Let your doctor make the diagnosis.

As I have noted earlier in this book, the first sign of chronic angina typically occurs when you are under unusual physical or emotional stress. In such situations, your heart beats faster and your blood pressure increases, and bloodflow through your coronary arteries must increase in response. If one or more of your arteries is substantially blocked, you may be unable to supply the required increase in bloodflow and your heart muscle will, in a sense, cry out for more blood. This 'cry' is manifested as chest pain. When the stress is removed (you stop running or reach the top of the stairs, for example), your heart rate and blood pressure return towards normal, your heart muscle requires less blood, and the chest pain goes away.

Although the plaque rupture leading to the obstruction may have occurred months or even years ago, it will not become apparent until you do an activity that requires a substantial increase in coronary bloodflow. Many of us who do not regularly do vigorous exercise will remain oblivious to a new obstruction. If we rush for a plane, shovel snow, move furniture, or experience unusual emotional stress, suddenly the heart muscle will require more bloodflow than can be supplied through the obstructed coronary artery, and chest pain will result. At rest or with mild exertion, the bloodflow will be adequate and chest pain will not be experienced.

In patients with the exertional symptoms described on page 240 or with a chest pain pattern that is atypical for angina, I perform a stress test (see page 210) to first establish whether the symptoms are due to a limitation of bloodflow. If that is the case, I then determine how much of the heart muscle is compromised and at what level of exercise capacity the symptoms and limitation of bloodflow occur. The earlier symptoms occur and the greater the amount of heart muscle affected, the more likely I am to proceed with an invasive approach. When exercise capacity is good and compromise of bloodflow is limited, the more likely I am to treat with medications and lifestyle interventions alone. For many people, this type of medical therapy can relieve angina and reverse the abnormalities seen on the stress test.

Is It a Stroke?

Many of us fear a stroke more than a heart attack because if we survive, we may be left with paralysis and a severely reduced quality of life. Each year, approximately 700,000 Americans and over 130,000 people in the UK suffer a stroke. Today more than 1 million American adults and 300,000 British adults have long-term disabilities as the result of a stroke.

You don't have to be one of those people. As with treating heart disease, aggressive risk-factor intervention can prevent strokes. The same medications and lifestyle therapies that can reduce the risk of having a heart attack can do the same for a stroke.

There are two different types of stroke: *haemorrhagic stroke* and *ischaemic stroke*. Haemorrhagic stroke is caused by the rupture of an artery and the release of blood into the brain. The major risk factor for haemorrhagic stroke is high blood pressure. An ischaemic stroke is caused by a sudden blockage of one of the arteries leading to the brain due to the rupture of a soft plaque and the resulting blood clot. Or it may be caused by a clot or atherosclerotic debris that has travelled to the brain from the heart or the vessels leading to the brain. Almost 90 per cent of strokes are ischaemic.

An ischaemic stroke is very similar to a heart attack, which is why some people refer to this type of stroke as a 'brain attack'. Therapies that reduce the risk of soft plaque rupture in the coronary arteries also reduce the risk of soft plaque rupture in the arteries leading to the brain.

If the clot blocks a small artery leading to the brain, the stroke may be so minor that the person is not aware of having had one. This is called a *silent stroke*. Silent strokes are quite common in older people and are believed to cause problems with memory and the ability to think. In a study of 5000 people 65 years of age and older, brain scans showed that 31 per cent had some stroke-related brain damage. Another 28 per cent had clear evidence of brain damage, even though they were not aware of having had a stroke or any stroke symptoms.

It's critical to know the symptoms of stroke so you can recognize when it's happening to you and get help. Stroke symptoms in both men and women include:

- Sudden weakness or numbness in the face, arm or leg on one side of the body

- A severe headache worse than anything you have ever experienced (this is most characteristic of a bleed into the brain)

- Slurred speech, loss of speech, and/or sudden blurring or loss of vision

- Dizziness, drowsiness or falls

You may experience one or more of these symptoms briefly and then go back to feeling normal. This is called a *transient ischaemic attack* (TIA). It is common to have several TIAs prior to having a stroke. If you think you have experienced a TIA, seek immediate medical attention.

For the most part, the same risk factors for heart disease apply to stroke. *Women, take note:* If you take oestrogen either in the form of oral contraceptives, the Patch, or hormone replacement therapy, you are at greater risk for stroke. Women who smoke and take birth control pills have a considerably greater risk of stroke (and heart attack) because each predisposes you to abnormal blood clot formation.

If you suspect that you are having a stroke, get medical attention immediately. Call 999 for an ambulance to take you to the hospital. If you are in the midst of having a stroke, the Accident and Emergency doctor may administer a drug to break up the clot to restore normal bloodflow to your brain. Drug therapy works best during the first 3 hours of a stroke and can make a real difference in terms of outcome. However, treatment once a stroke has occurred is quite limited. The best strategy is prevention.

Fortunately, the simple, painless, noninvasive carotid ultrasound test we discussed in Step 3 can be performed to detect the buildup of plaque in the carotid arteries, which carry blood to your brain. Plaque buildup in the carotids generally occurs later than it does in the coronary arteries; however, atherosclerosis in the carotids can still be seen years before it could lead to a stroke. If you have cardiac risk factors and a family history of heart disease or stroke, then a screening carotid ultrasound can be very helpful. If atherosclerosis is detected, its response to therapy and lifestyle changes can be monitored. Discuss your risk of stroke and the potential benefits of a carotid ultrasound with your doctor. With the information obtained from the ultrasound, your doctor can decide if you need to make any changes in your lifestyle or take medications such as a statin drug, a blood pressure-lowering drug, or a blood thinner to prevent a stroke.

Helpful Resources

For more information on heart disease and stroke, diet, exercise, stopping smoking and a healthy lifestyle, contact:

UK
British Heart Foundation
14 Fitzhardinge Street
London W1H 6DH
Tel: 020 7935 0185
Information line: 0845 070 8070
www.bhf.org.uk

British Lung Foundation
73-75 Goswell Road
London EC1V 7ER
Helpline: 0845 850 5020
www.blf-uk.org

HEART UK
7 North Road
Maidenhead
Berkshire SL6 1PE
Tel: 01628 628638
Helpline: 0845 450 5988
Email: *ask@heartuk.org.uk*
www.heartuk.org.uk

NHS Direct
Tel: 0845 4647
www.nhsdirect.nhs.uk

NHS Smoking helpline: 0800 169 0169
www.givingupsmoking.co.uk
(or contact your GP for help, information and advice on stopping smoking)

The Stroke Association
Stroke Information Service
240 City Road
London EC1V 2PR
Helpline: 0845 303 3100
Email: *info@stroke.org.uk*
www.stroke.org.uk

For more information on diabetes, contact:

Diabetes UK
Diabetes UK Central Office
Macleod House
10 Parkway
London NW1 7AA
Tel: 020 7424 1000
Diabetes Careline: 0845 120 2960
Email: *info@diabetes.org.uk*
www.diabetes.org.uk

To find a local CPR/emergency first aid training course in your area, contact:

British Red Cross
www.redcross.org.uk

St John Ambulance
www.sja.org.uk

or your local NHS Trust

AUSTRALIA
Heart Foundation
Level 3, 80 William Street
Sydney NSW 2011
Tel: (02) 9219 2444
Fax: (02) 9219 2424
Email: *heartline@heartfoundation.com.au*

National Stroke Foundation
Level 8, 99 Queen Street
Melbourne VIC 3000
Tel: (03) 9670 1000
Fax: (03) 9670 9300
www.strokefoundation.com.au

Quit Now Australia
Freecall: 131 848
Tel: (02) 6289 1555
Email: *quitnow@health.gov.au*
www.quitnow.info.au
(for advice on stopping smoking)

Quit Victoria
PO Box 888
Carlton VIC 3053
Tel: (03) 9663 7777
Fax: (03) 9635 5510
www.quit.org.au
(for advice on stopping smoking)

St John Ambulance Australia
Cnr Canberra Ave and Dominion Crt
Forrest ACT 2603
PO Box 3895
Manuka ACT 2603
Tel: (02) 6295 3777
Fax: (02) 6239 6321
Email: *enquiries@stjohn.org.au*
(to find a CPR/emergency first aid
training course)

SELECTED BIBLIOGRAPHY

CHAPTER 1
You Don't Have to Have a Heart Attack!

Aaron HJ. *Treatment of Coronary Artery Disease: What Does Rationing Do?* Policy Brief #148. Washington, DC: The Brookings Institution, 2005.

Agatston A. *The South Beach Diet*. Emmaus, Pennsylvania: Rodale, 2003.

Agatston AS, Janowitz WR, et al. Quantification of coronary artery calcium using ultrafast computed tomography. *J Am Coll Cardiol* 1990;15(4):827–832.

Banks J, Marmot M, et al. Disease and disadvantage in the United States and in England. *JAMA* 2006;295(17):2037–2045.

Bloomgarden ZT. Type 2 diabetes in the young. *Diabetes Care* 2004;27(4):998–1010.

Lucas FL, DeLorenzo MA, et al. Temporal trends in the utilization of diagnostic testing and treatments for cardiovascular disease in the United States, 1993–2001. *Circulation* 2006;113(3):374–379.

Ma J, Sehgal NL, et al. National trends in statin use by coronary heart disease risk category. *PLoS Med* 2005;2(5):e123.

McBride P, Schrott HG, et al. Primary care practice adherence to National Cholesterol Education Program guidelines for patients with coronary heart disease. *Arch Intern Med* 1998;158(11):1238–1244.

Newsom SW. Pioneers in infection control – Joseph Lister. *J Hosp Infect* 2003;55(4): 246–253.

Sueta CA, Chowdhury M, et al. Analysis of the degree of undertreatment of hyperlipidemia and congestive heart failure secondary to coronary artery disease. *Am J Cardiol* 1999;83(9):1303–1307.

Thom T, Haase N, et al. Heart disease and stroke statistics – 2006 update: A report from the American Heart Association Statistics Committee and Stroke Statistics Subcommittee. *Circulation* 2006;113(6):e85–e151.

CHAPTER 2
Why 'Perfectly Healthy' People Get Heart Attacks

Corti R, Fuster V, et al. Pathogenetic concepts of acute coronary syndromes. *J Am Coll Cardiol* 2003;41(4 Suppl S):7S–14S.

Davies MJ. Acute coronary thrombosis – The role of plaque disruption and its initiation and prevention. *Eur Heart J* 1995;16 Suppl L:3–7.

DeWood MA, Spores J, et al. Prevalence of total coronary occlusion during the early hours of transmural myocardial infarction. *N Engl J Med* 1980;303(16):897–902.

Falk E. Pathogenesis of atherosclerosis. *J Am Coll Cardiol* 2006;47(8 Suppl):C7–C12.

Fuster V, Moreno PR, et al. Atherothrombosis and high-risk plaque: Part I: Evolving concepts. *J Am Coll Cardiol* 2005;46(6):937–954.

Heil M, Schaper W. Pathophysiology of collateral development. *Coron Artery Dis* 2004;15(7):373–378.

King SB 3rd. Angioplasty from bench to bedside to bench. *Circulation* 1996;93(9): 1621–1622.

Koerselman J, van der Graaf Y, et al. Coronary collaterals: An important and underexposed aspect of coronary artery disease. *Circulation* 2003;107(19):2507–2511.

Viles-Gonzalez JF, Fuster V, et al. Atherothrombosis: A widespread disease with unpredictable and life-threatening consequences. *Eur Heart J* 2004;25(14):1197–1207.

CHAPTER 3
You May Be at Risk and What You Can Do about It

Birtcher KK, Ballantyne CM. Cardiology patient page. Measurement of cholesterol: A patient perspective. *Circulation* 2004;110(11):e296–e297.

Black PH, Garbutt LD. Stress, inflammation and cardiovascular disease. *J Psychosom Res* 2002;52(1):1–23.

Blake GJ, Rifai N, et al. Blood pressure, C-reactive protein, and risk of future cardiovascular events. *Circulation* 2003;108(24):2993–2999.

Bonaa KH, Njolstad I, et al. Homocysteine lowering and cardiovascular events after acute myocardial infarction. *N Engl J Med* 2006;354(15):1578–1588.

Bottiglieri T. Homocysteine and folate metabolism in depression. *Prog Neuropsychopharmacol Biol Psychiatry* 2005;29(7):1103–1112.

Chobanian AV, Bakris GL, et al. Seventh report of the Joint National Committee on Prevention, Detection, Evaluation, and Treatment of High Blood Pressure. *Hypertension* 2003;42(6):1206–1252.

Expert Panel on Detection, Evaluation, and Treatment of High Blood Cholesterol in Adults. Executive summary of the Third Report of the National Cholesterol Education Program (NCEP) Expert Panel on Detection, Evaluation, and Treatment of High Blood Cholesterol in Adults (Adult Treatment Panel III). *JAMA* 2001;285(19):2486–2497.

Ganji V, Kafai MR. Frequent consumption of milk, yogurt, cold breakfast cereals, peppers, and cruciferous vegetables and intakes of dietary folate and riboflavin but not vitamins B-12 and B-6 are inversely associated with serum total homocysteine concentrations in the US population. *Am J Clin Nutr* 2004;80(6):1500–1507.

Gaziano JM, Hennekens CH, et al. Fasting triglycerides, high-density lipoprotein, and risk of myocardial infarction. *Circulation* 1997;96(8):2520–2525.

Grundy SM, Cleeman JI, et al. Implications of recent clinical trials for the National Cholesterol Education Program Adult Treatment Panel III guidelines. *Circulation* 2004;110(2):227–239.

Heilbronn LK, Noakes M, et al. Energy restriction and weight loss on very low-fat diets reduce C-reactive protein concentrations in obese, healthy women. *Ateriosder Throm Vas Biol* 2001;21(16):968–970.

Joint British Societies' Guidelines on Prevention of Cardiovascular Disease in Clinical Practice. *Heart* 2005; 91: Supplement J.

Kang MG, Koh SB, et al. Association between job stress on heart rate variability and metabolic syndrome in shipyard male workers. *Yonsei Med J* 2004;45(5):838–846.

Kang MG, Koh SB, et al. Job stress and cardiovascular risk factors in male workers. *Prev Med* 2005;40(5):583–588.

Kannel WB, Dawber TR, et al. Factors of risk in the development of coronary heart disease – Six year follow-up experience: The Framingham Study. *Ann Intern Med* 1961;55:33–50.

Kris-Etherton PM, Harris WS, et al. Fish consumption, fish oil, omega-3 fatty acids, and cardiovascular disease. *Circulation* 2002;106(21):2747–2757.

Lightwood J. Estimating the impact of secondhand smoke. Abstract presented at the American Heart Association Seventh Scientific Forum on Quality of Care and Outcomes Research in Cardiovascular Disease and Stroke, Washington, DC, May 7–9, 2006.

Lonn E, Yusuf S, et al. Homocysteine lowering with folic acid and B vitamins in vascular disease. *N Engl J Med* 2006;354(15):1567–1577.

Maeda K, Noguchi Y, et al. The effects of cessation from cigarette smoking on the lipid and lipoprotein profiles: a meta-analysis. *Prev Med* 2003;37(4):283–290.

Mehta NJ, Khan IA. Cardiology's 10 greatest discoveries of the 20th century. *Tex Heart Inst J* 2002;29(3):164–171.

Moffat RJ. Effects of cessation of smoking on serum lipids and high-density lipoprotein cholesterol. *Atherosclerosis* 1988;74(1–2):85–89.

Mosca L, Edelman D, et al. Waist circumference predicts cardiometabolic and global Framingham risk among women screened during National Woman's Heart Day. *J Womens Health* 2006;15(1):24–34.

Murabito JM, Pencina MJ, et al. Sibling cardiovascular disease as a risk factor for cardiovascular disease in middle-aged adults. *JAMA* 2005;294(24):3117–3123.

Nabel EG. Cardiovascular disease. *N Engl J Med* 2003;349(1):60–72.

Nissen SE, Tuzcu EM, et al. Effect of antihypertensive agents on cardiovascular events in patients with coronary disease and normal blood pressure: The CAMELOT study: A randomized controlled trial. *JAMA* 2004;292(18):2217–2225.

Qureshi AI, Suri MF, et al. Is prehypertension a risk factor for cardiovascular diseases? *Stroke* 2005;36(9):1859–1863.

Ridker PM, Cannon CP, et al. C-reactive protein levels and outcomes after statin therapy. *N Engl J Med* 2005;352(1):20–28.

Ridker PM, Cushman M, et al. Inflammation, aspirin and the risk of cardiovascular disease in apparently healthy men. *N Engl J Med* 1997;336(14):973–979.

Ridker PM, Hennekens CH, et al. C-reactive protein and other markers of inflammation in the prediction of cardiovascular disease in women. *N Engl J Med* 2000;342(12):836–843.

Salpeter SR, Walsh JM, et al. Brief report: Coronary heart disease events associated with hormone therapy in younger and older women. A meta-analysis. *J Gen Intern Med* 2006;21(4):363–366.

Selhub J. The many facets of hyperhomocysteinemia: Studies from the Framingham cohorts. *J Nutr* 2006;136(6 Suppl):1726S–1730S.

Selhub J, Jacques PF, et al. Association between plasma homocysteine concentrations and extracranial carotid-artery stenosis. *N Engl J Med* 1995;332(5):286–291.

Tanne D, Medalie JH, et al. Body fat distribution and long-term risk of stroke mortality. *Stroke* 2005;36(5):1021–1025.

Tenerz A, Lonnberg I, et al. Myocardial infarction and prevalence of diabetes mellitus. Is increased casual blood glucose at admission a reliable criterion for the diagnosis of diabetes? *Eur Heart J* 2001;22(13):1102–1110.

Toth PP. Cardiology patient page. The 'good cholesterol': High-density lipoprotein. *Circulation* 2005;111(5):e89–e91.

Venugopal SK, Devaraj S, et al. Demonstration that C-reactive protein decreases eNOS expression and bioactivity in human aortic endothelial cells. *Circulation* 2002;106(12):1439–1441.

Whiteley L, Padmanabhan S, et al. Should diabetes be considered a coronary heart disease risk equivalent? Results from 25 years of follow-up in the Renfrew and Paisley Survey. *Diabetes Care* 2005;28(7):1588–1593.

Willingham SA, Kilpatrick ES. Evidence of gender bias when applying the new diagnostic criteria for myocardial infarction. *Heart* 2005;91(2):237–238.

Yusuf S, Hawken S, et al. Effect of potentially modifiable risk factors associated with myocardial infarction in 52 countries (the INTERHEART study): Case-control study. *Lancet* 2004;364(9438):937–952.

Zerwic JJ, King KB, et al. Perceptions of patients with cardiovascular disease about the causes of coronary artery disease. *Heart Lung* 1997;26(2):92–98.

CHAPTER 4
What Size Is Your Cholesterol?

Lewis GF, Rader DJ. New insights into the regulation of HDL metabolism and reverse cholesterol transport. *Circ Res* 2005;96(12):1221–1232.

McNagny SE, Wenger NK, et al. Personal use of postmenopausal hormone replacement therapy by women physicians in the United States. *Ann Intern Med* 1997;127(12):1093–1096.

Mendelsohn ME, Karas RH. The protective effects of estrogen on the cardiovascular system. *N Engl J Med* 1999;340(23):1801–1811.

Rossouw JE, Anderson GL, et al. Risks and benefits of estrogen plus progestin in healthy postmenopausal women: Principal results from the Women's Health Initiative randomized controlled trial. *JAMA* 2002;288(3):321–333.

Steinberg D. Thematic review series: The pathogenesis of atherosclerosis. An interpretive history of the cholesterol controversy: Part I. *J Lipid Res* 2004;45(9):1583–1593.

Steinberg D. Thematic review series: The pathogenesis of atherosclerosis. An interpretive history of the cholesterol controversy: Part II: The early evidence linking hypercholesterolemia to coronary disease in humans. *J Lipid Res* 2005;46(2):179–190.

Superko HR, Tucker L. *Before the Heart Attacks*. Emmaus, Pennsylvania: Rodale, 2003.

CHAPTER 5
What Your Waistline Says about Your Heart

Cordain L. Cereal grains: Humanity's double-edged sword. *World Rev Nutr Diet* 1999;84:19–73.

Eaton SB, Konner M. Paleolithic nutrition. A consideration of its nature and current implications. *N Engl J Med* 1985;312(5):283–289.

Eaton SB, Konner M, et al. Stone agers in the fast lane: Chronic degenerative diseases in evolutionary perspective. *Am J Med* 1988;84(4):739–749.

Esposito K, Marfella R, et al. Effect of a Mediterranean-style diet on endothelial dysfunction and markers of vascular inflammation in the metabolic syndrome: A randomized trial. *JAMA* 2004;292(12):1440–1446.

Keys A. Coronary heart disease in seven countries. *Circulation* 1970;41:1–211.

Klein S, Fontana L, et al. Absence of an effect of liposuction on insulin action and risk factors for coronary heart disease. *N Engl J Med* 2004;350(25):2549–2557.

Knowler WC, Pettitt DJ, et al. Obesity in the Pima Indians: Its magnitude and relationship with diabetes. *Am J Clin Nutr* 1991;53(6 Suppl):1543S–1551S.

Kriketos AD, Greenfield JR, et al. Inflammation, insulin resistance, and adiposity: A study of first-degree relatives of type 2 diabetic subjects. *Diabetes Care* 2004;27(8):2033–2040.

Reaven GM. Syndrome X: 6 years later. *J Intern Med Suppl* 1994;736:13–22.

Rexrode KM, Carey VJ, et al. Abdominal adiposity and coronary heart disease in women. *JAMA* 1998;280(21):1843–1848.

Ross R. Atherosclerosis – An inflammatory disease. *N Engl J Med* 1999;340(2):115–126.

Seidell JC, Bjorntorp P, et al. Visceral fat accumulation in men is positively associated with insulin, glucose, and C-peptide levels, but negatively with testosterone levels. *Metabolism* 1990;39(9):897–901.

Simopoulos AP. Evolutionary aspects of diet, essential fatty acids and cardiovascular disease. *Eur Heart J Suppl* 2001;3(Suppl D):D8–D21.

Tchernof A, Calles-Escandon J, et al. Menopause, central body fatness, and insulin resistance: Effects of hormone-replacement therapy. *Coron Artery Dis* 1998;9(8):503–511.

Van Oijen M, Witteman JC, et al. Fibrinogen is associated with an increased risk of Alzheimer disease and vascular dementia. *Stroke* 2005;36(12):2637–2641.

Vine AK, Stader J, et al. Biomarkers of cardiovascular disease as risk factors for age-related macular degeneration. *Ophthalmology* 2005;112(12):2076–2080.

Zimmet P. Global and societal implications of the diabetes epidemic. *Nature* 2001;414: 782–787.

CHAPTER 6
Every Picture Tells a Story

Agatston AS, Janowitz WR, et al. Quantification of coronary artery calcium using ultrafast computed tomography. *J Am Coll Cardiol* 1990;15(4):827–832.

Akosah KO, Schaper A, et al. Preventing myocardial infarction in the young adult in the first place: How do the National Cholesterol Education Panel III guidelines perform? *J Am Coll Cardiol* 2003;41(9):1475–1479.

Arad Y, Goodman KJ, et al. Coronary calcification, coronary disease risk factors, C-reactive protein, and atherosclerotic cardiovascular disease events: The St. Francis Heart Study. *J Am Coll Cardiol* 2005;46(1):158–165.

Berenson GS. Bogalusa Heart Study: A long-term community study of a rural biracial (black/white) population. *Am J Med Sci* 2001;322(5):293–300.

Berger JS, Roncaglioni MC, et al. Aspirin for the primary prevention of cardiovascular events in women and men: A sex-specific meta-analysis of randomized controlled trials. *JAMA* 2006;295(3):306–313.

Blackburn DF, Dobson RT, et al. Adherence to statins, beta-blockers and angiotensin-converting enzyme inhibitors following a first cardiovascular event: A retrospective cohort study. *Can J Cardiol* 2005;21(6):485–488.

Budoff MJ, Georgiou D, et al. Ultrafast computed tomography as a diagnostic modality in the detection of coronary artery disease: A multicenter study. *Circulation* 1996;93(5):898–904.

Coles DR, Smail MA, et al. Comparison of radiation doses from multislice computed tomography coronary angiography and conventional diagnostic angiography. *J Am Coll Cardiol* 2006;47(9):1840–1845.

Greenland P, LaBree L, et al. Coronary artery calcium score combined with Framingham score for risk prediction in asymptomatic individuals. *JAMA* 2004;291(2):210–215.

Hecht HS. Practice guidelines for electron beam tomography: A report of the Society of Atherosclerosis Imaging. *Am J Cardiol* 2000;86(6):705–706.

Hecht HS, Budoff MJ, et al. Coronary artery calcium scanning: Clinical paradigms for cardiac risk assessment and treatment. *Am Heart J* 2006;151(6):1139–1146.

Hoff JA, Chomka EV, et al. Age and gender distributions of coronary artery calcium detected by electron beam tomography in 35,246 adults. *Am J Cardiol* 2001;87(12):1335–1339.

Janowitz WR, Agatston AS, et al. Comparison of serial quantitative evaluation of calcified coronary artery plaque by ultrafast computed tomography in persons with and without obstructive coronary artery disease. *Am J Cardiol* 1991;68(1):1–6.

Janowitz WR, Agatston AS, et al. Differences in prevalence and extent of coronary artery calcium detected by ultrafast computed tomography in asymptomatic men and women. *Am J Cardiol* 1993;72(3):247–254.

Kalia NK, Miller LG, et al. Visualizing coronary calcium is associated with improvements in adherence to statin therapy. *Atherosclerosis* 2006;185(2):394–399.

Kondos GT, Hoff JA, et al. Electron beam tomography coronary artery calcium and cardiac events. A 37-month follow-up of 5635 initially asymptomatic low- to intermediate-risk adults. *Circulation* 2003;107(20):2571–2576.

Kulkarni SP, Alexander KP, et al. Long-term adherence with cardiovascular drug regimens. *Am Heart J* 2006;151(1):185–191.

Nicholls SJ, Tuzcu EM. Relationship between cardiovascular risk factors and atherosclerotic disease burden measured by intravascular ultrasound. *J Am Coll Cardiol* 2006;47(10):1967–1975.

O'Malley PG, Taylor AJ, et al. Prognostic value of coronary electron-beam computed tomography for coronary heart disease events in asymptomatic populations. *Am J Cardiol* 2000;85(8):945–948.

Raggi P, Callister TQ, et al. Identification of patients at increased risk of first unheralded acute myocardial infarction by electron beam computed tomography. *Circulation* 2000;101(8):850–855.

Rumberger JA, Schwartz RS, et al. Relation of coronary calcium determined by electron beam computed tomography and lumen narrowing determined by autopsy. *Am J Cardiol* 1994;73(16):1169–1173.

Rumberger JA, Simons DB, et al. Coronary artery calcium area by electron beam computed tomography and coronary atherosclerotic plaque area: A histopathologic correlative study. *Circulation* 1995;92(8):2157–2162.

Schartl M, Bocksch W, et al. Effects of lipid-lowering therapy on coronary artery remodeling. *Coron Artery Dis* 2004;15(1):45–51.

Schoenhagen P, Tuzcu EM, et al. Determinants of arterial wall remodeling during lipid-lowering therapy: Serial intravascular ultrasound observations from the Reversal of Atherosclerosis with Aggressive Lipid Lowering Therapy (REVERSAL) trial. *Circulation* 2006;113(24):2826–2834.

Shaw LJ, Raggi P, et al. Prognostic value of cardiac risk factors and coronary artery calcium screening for all-cause mortality. *Radiology* 2003;228(3):826–833.

CHAPTER 7
Should You Be Taking Heart Medications?

Blake GJ, Ridker PM. Are statins anti-inflammatory? *Curr Control Trials Cardiovasc Med* 2000;1(3):161–165.

Blumenthal RS, Kapur NK. Can a potent statin actually regress coronary atherosclerosis? *JAMA* 2006;295(13):1583–1584.

Cannon CP, Braunwald E, et al. Intensive versus moderate lipid lowering with statins after acute coronary syndromes. *N Engl J Med* 2004;350(15):1495–1504.

Corti R, Fuster V. Should standard medical therapy for angina include a statin? *Clin Cardiol* 2004;27(10):547–551.

Dagenais GR, Yusuf S, et al. Effects of ramipril on coronary events in high-risk persons: Results of the Heart Outcomes Prevention Evaluation Study. *Circulation* 2001;104(5): 522–526.

Davignon J. Beneficial cardiovascular pleiotropic effects of statins. *Circulation* 2004;109 (23 Suppl 1):III39–III43.

Downs JR, Clearfield M, et al. Primary prevention of acute coronary events with lovastatin in men and women with average cholesterol levels: Results of AFCAPS/TexCAPS. *JAMA* 1998;279(20):1615–1622.

Fonarow GC, Wright RS, et al. Effect of statin use within the first 24 hours of admission for acute myocardial infarction on early morbidity and mortality. *Am J Cardiol* 2005;96(5):611–616.

Ford ES, Mokdad AH, et al. Serum total cholesterol concentrations and awareness, treatment, and control of hypercholesterolemia among US adults: Findings from the National Health and Nutrition Examination Survey, 1999 to 2000. *Circulation* 2003;107(17):2185–2189.

Frick MH, Elo O, et al. Helsinki Heart Study: Primary-prevention trial with gemfibrozil in middle-aged men with dyslipidemia. Safety of treatment, changes in risk factors, and incidence of coronary heart disease. *N Engl J Med* 1987;317(20):1237–1245.

Frolkis JP. Should one routinely screen for lipoprotein(a)? *Cleve Clin J Med* 1999;66(8): 465–468.

Frolkis JP, Zyzanski SJ, et al. Physician noncompliance with the 1993 National Cholesterol Education Program (NCEP-ATPII) guidelines. *Circulation* 1998;98(9):851–855.

Heart Protection Study Collaborative Group. MRC/BHF Heart Protection Study of cholesterol lowering with simvastatin in 20,536 high-risk individuals: A randomised placebo-controlled trial. *Lancet* 2002;360(9326):7–22.

Joint British Societies' Guidelines on Prevention of Cardiovascular Disease in Clinical Practice. *Heart* 2005; 91: Supplement J.

LaRosa JC, Grundy SM, et al. Intensive lipid lowering with atorvastatin in patients with stable coronary disease. *N Engl J Med* 2005;352(14):1425–1435.

The Lipid Research Clinics Coronary Primary Prevention Trial results. I. Reduction in incidence of coronary heart disease. *JAMA* 1984;251:351–364.

Narayan KM, Mensah GA, et al. Combination pharmacotherapy for cardiovascular disease prevention: Threat or opportunity for public health? *Am J Prev Med* 2005;29 (5 Suppl 1):134–138.

Nissen SE, Tuzcu EM, et al. Effect of intensive compared with moderate lipid-lowering therapy on progression of coronary atherosclerosis: A randomized controlled trial. *JAMA* 2004;291(9):1071–1080.

O'Keefe JH Jr, Cordain L, et al. Coronary artery disease prognosis and C-reactive protein levels improve in proportion to percent lowering of low-density lipoprotein. *Am J Cardiol* 2006;98(1):135–139.

Randomised trial of cholesterol lowering in 4444 patients with coronary heart disease: the Scandinavian Simvastatin Survival Study (4S). *Lancet* 1994;344(8934):1383–1389.

Rouleau J. Improved outcome after acute coronary syndromes with an intensive versus standard lipid-lowering regimen: Results from the Pravastatin or Atorvastatin Evaluation and Infection Therapy–Thrombolysis in Myocardial Infarction 22 (PROVE-IT–TIMI 22) trial. *Am J Med* 2005;118 Suppl 12A:28–35.

Rubins HB, Robins SJ, et al. Gemfibrozil for the secondary prevention of coronary heart disease in men with low levels of high-density lipoprotein cholesterol. *N.Engl J Med* 1999;341(6):410–418.

Schaefer EJ, McNamara JR, et al. Effects of atorvastatin versus other statins on fasting and postprandial C-reactive protein and lipoprotein-associated phospholipase A2 in patients with coronary heart disease versus control subjects. *Am J Cardiol* 2005;95:1025–1032.

Scirica BM, Cannon CP. Treatment of elevated cholesterol. *Circulation* 2005;111(21): e360–e363.

Shepherd J, Cobbe SM, et al. Prevention of coronary heart disease with pravastatin in men with hypercholesterolemia. *N Engl J Med* 1995;333(20):1301–1307.

Wald NJ, Law MR. A strategy to reduce cardiovascular disease by more than 80%. *BMJ* 2003;326(7404):1419.

Whincup PH, Emberson JR, et al. Low prevalence of lipid lowering drug use in older men with established coronary heart disease. *Heart* 2002;88(1):25–29.

Wong ND, Budoff MJ, et al. Coronary calcium and cardiovascular event risk: Evaluation by age- and sex-specific quartiles. *Am Heart J* 2002;143(3):456–459.

CHAPTER 8

Is This Procedure Really Necessary?

Alderman EL, Bourassa MG, et al. Ten-year follow-up of survival and myocardial infarction in the randomized Coronary Artery Surgery Study. *Circulation* 1990;82(5):1629–1646.

Bucher HC, Hengstler P, et al. Percutaneous transluminal coronary angioplasty versus medical treatment for non-acute coronary heart disease: Meta-analysis of randomised controlled trials. *BMJ* 2000;321(7253):73–77.

Davies JR, Rudd JH, et al. Molecular and metabolic imaging of atherosclerosis. *J Nucl Med* 2004;45(11):1898–1907.

Katritsis DG, Ioannidis JP. Percutaneous coronary intervention versus conservative therapy in nonacute coronary artery disease: A meta-analysis. *Circulation* 2005;111(22):2906–2912.

McFalls EO, Ward HB, et al. Coronary-artery revascularization before elective major vascular surgery. *N Engl J Med* 2004;351(27):2795–2804.

Meier B. The first patient to undergo coronary angioplasty – 23-year follow-up. *N Engl J Med* 2001;344(2):144–145.

Morrison DA, Sacks J. Balancing benefit against risk in the choice of therapy for coronary artery disease. Lesson from prospective, randomized, clinical trials of percutaneous coronary intervention and coronary artery bypass graft surgery. *Minerva Cardioangiol* 2003;51(5):585–597.

Pitt B, Waters D, et al. Aggressive lipid-lowering therapy compared with angioplasty in stable coronary artery disease. *N Engl J Med* 1999;341(2):70–76.

Rihal CS, Raco DL, et al. Indications for coronary artery bypass surgery and percutaneous coronary intervention in chronic stable angina: Review of the evidence and methodological considerations. *Circulation* 2003;108(20):2439–2445.

RITA-2 Trial Participants. Coronary angioplasty versus medical therapy for angina: The second Randomised Intervention Treatment of Angina (RITA-2) trial. *Lancet* 1997;350(9076):461–468.

STEP 1

Following the Principles of the South Beach Diet

Agatston A. *The South Beach Diet*. Emmaus, Pennsylvania: Rodale, 2003.

Alonso A, Beunza JJ, et al. Low-fat dairy consumption and reduced risk of hypertension: The Seguimiento Universidad de Navarra (SUN) Cohort. *Am J Clin Nutr* 2005;82(5):972–979.

Anderson JW, Hanna TJ, et al. Whole grain foods and heart disease risk. *J Am Coll Nutr* 2000;19(3 Suppl):291S–299S.

Anderson KJ, Teuber SS, et al. Walnut polyphenolics inhibit in vitro human plasma and LDL oxidation. *J Nutr* 2001;131(11):2837–2842.

Appel LJ, Sacks FM, et al. The effects of protein, monounsaturated fat, and carbohydrate intake on blood pressure and serum lipids: Results of the OmniHeart randomized trial. *JAMA* 2005;294(19):2455–2464.

Aravanis C, Corcondilas A, et al. Coronary heart disease in seven countries. IX. The Greek islands of Crete and Corfu. *Circulation* 1970;41(4 Suppl):I88–I100.

Aude YW, Agatston AS, et al. The National Cholesterol Education Program diet vs a diet lower in carbohydrates and higher in protein and monounsaturated fat: A randomized trial. *Arch Intern Med* 2004;164(19):2141–2146.

Aviram M, Rosenblat M. Pomegranate juice consumption for 3 years by patients with carotid artery stenosis reduces common carotid intima-media thickness, blood pressure and LDL oxidation. *Clin Nutr* 2004;23(3):423–433.

Bazzano LA, He J, et al. Legume consumption and the risk of coronary heart disease in US men and women: NHANES I epidemiologic follow-up study. *Arch Intern Med* 2001;161(21):2573–2578.

Blackburn H, Taylor HL, et al. Coronary heart disease in seven countries. XVI. The electrocardiogram in prediction of five-year coronary heart disease incidence among men aged forty through fifty-nine. *Circulation* 1970;41(4 Suppl):I154–I161.

Brand-Miller J. Optimizing the cardiovascular outcomes of weight loss. *Am J Clin Nutr* 2005;81(5):949–950.

De Lorgeril M, Renaud S, et al. Mediterranean alpha-linolenic acid-rich diet in secondary prevention of coronary heart disease. *Lancet* 1994;343(8911):1454–1459.

Diebolt M, Bucher B, et al. Wine polyphenols decrease blood pressure, improve NO vasodilatation, and induce gene expression. *Hypertension* 2001;38(2):159–165.

Ebbeling CB, Leidig MM, et al. Effects of an ad libitum low-glycemic load diet on cardiovascular disease risk factors in obese young adults. *Am J Clin Nutr* 2005;81(5):976–982.

FDA Authorizes New Coronary Heart Disease Health Claim for Plant Sterol and Plant Stanol Esters. FDA Talk Paper #T00-40. Rockville, Maryland: Food and Drug Administration, 2000.

Grassi D, Lippi C, et al. Short-term administration of dark chocolate is followed by a significant increase in insulin sensitivity and a decrease in blood pressure in healthy persons. *Am J Clin Nutr* 2005;81(3):611–614.

Howard BV, Van Horn L, et al. Low-fat dietary pattern and risk of cardiovascular disease: The Women's Health Initiative Randomized Controlled Dietary Modification Trial. *JAMA* 2006;295(6):655–666.

Hu FB, Stampfer MJ. Nut consumption and risk of coronary heart disease: A review of epidemiological evidence. *Curr Atheroscler Report* 1999;1(3):204–209.

Liu L, Zubik L, et al. The antiatherogenic potential of oat phenolic compounds. *Atherosclerosis* 2004;175(1):39–49.

Liu RH. Health benefits of fruit and vegetables are from additive and synergistic combinations of phytochemicals. *Am J Clin Nutr* 2003;78(3 Suppl):517S–520S.

Ludwig DS, Pereira MA, et al. Dietary fiber, weight gain, and cardiovascular disease risk factors in young adults. *JAMA* 1999;282(16):1539–1546.

Masella R, Giovannini C, et al. Effects of dietary virgin olive oil phenols on low density lipoprotein oxidation in hyperlipidemic patients. *Lipids* 2001;36(11):1195–1202.

Miller HE, Rigelhof F, et al. Antioxidant content of whole grain breakfast cereals, fruits and vegetables. *J Am Coll Nutr* 2000;19(3 Suppl):312S–319S.

Nie L, Wise ML, et al. Avenanthramide, a polyphenol from oats, inhibits vascular smooth muscle cell proliferation and enhances nitric oxide production. *Atherosclerosis* 2006;186(2):260–266.

Ohmori R, Iwamoto T, et al. Antioxidant activity of various teas against free radicals and LDL oxidation. *Lipids* 2005;40(8):849–853.

O'Keefe JH Jr, Harris WS. From Inuit to implementation: Omega 3 fatty acids come of age. *Mayo Clin Proc* 2000;75(6):607–614.

Olson ER, Naugle JE, et al. Inhibition of cardiac fibroblast proliferation and myofibroblast differentiation by resveratrol. *Am J Physiol Heart Circ Physiol* 2005;288(3):H1131–H1138.

Pereira MS, O'Reilly E, et al. Dietary fiber and risk of coronary heart disease: A pooled analysis of cohort studies. *Arch Intern Med* 2004;164(4):370–376.

Roberts WG, Gordon MH. Determination of the total antioxidant activity of fruits and vegetables by a liposome assay. *J Agric Food Chem* 2003;51(5):1486–1493.

Robitaille J, Fontaine-Bisson B, et al. Effect of an oat bran-rich supplement on the metabolic profile of overweight premenopausal women. *Ann Nutr Metab* 2005;49(3): 141–148.

Ruf JC. Overview of epidemiological studies on wine, health and mortality. *Drugs Exp Clin Res* 2003;29(5–6):173–179.

Rumpler W, Seale J, et al. Oolong tea increases metabolic rate and fat oxidation in men. *J Nutr* 2001;131(11):2848–2852.

Sahyoun NR, Jacques PF, et al. Whole-grain intake is inversely associated with the metabolic syndrome and mortality in older adults. *Am J Clin Nutr* 2006;83(1):124–131.

Shimada K, Kawarabayashi T, et al. Oolong tea increases plasma adiponectin levels and low-density lipoprotein particle size in patients with coronary artery disease. *Diabetes Res Clin Pract* 2004;65(3):227–234.

Sumner MD, Elliot-Eller M, et al. Effects of pomegranate juice consumption on myocardial perfusion in patients with coronary heart disease. *Am J Cardiol* 2005;96(6): 810–814.

Sung H, Min WK, et al. The effects of green tea ingestion over four weeks on atherosclerotic markers. *Ann Clin Biochem* 2005;42(Pt 4):292–297.

Tsang C, Higgins S, et al. The influence of moderate red wine consumption on antioxidant status and indices of oxidative stress associated with CHD in healthy volunteers. *Br J Nutr* 2005;93(2):233–240.

Van der Gaag MS, van Tol A, et al. Alcohol consumption stimulates early steps in reverse cholesterol transport. *J Lipid Res* 2001;42(12):2077–2083.

Whelton SP, Hyre AD, et al. Effect of dietary fiber intake on blood pressure: A meta-analysis of randomized, controlled clinical trials. *J Hypertens* 2005;23(3):475–481.

Wu JM, Wang ZR, et al. Mechanism of cardioprotection by resveratrol, a phenolic antioxidant present in red wine (review). *Int J Mol Med* 2001;8(1):3–17.

Wu X, Beecher GR, et al. Lipophilic and hydrophilic antioxidant capacities of common foods in the United States. *J Agric Food Chem* 2004;52(12):4026–4037.

Zhao G, Etherton TD, et al. Dietary alpha-linolenic acid reduces inflammatory and lipid cardiovascular risk factors in hypercholesterolemic men and women. *J Nutr* 2004;134(11):2991–2997.

STEP 2

The South Beach Heart Workout

Baster T, Baster-Brooks C. Exercise and hypertension. *Aust Fam Physician* 2005;34(6):419–424.

Blair SN, Kampert JB, et al. Influences of cardiorespiratory fitness and other precursors on cardiovascular disease and all-cause mortality in men and women. *JAMA* 1996;276(3):205–210.

Brown SG, Rhodes RE. Relationships among dog ownership and leisure time walking in Western Canadian adults. *Am J Prev Med* 2006;30(2):131–136.

Capuano CA. Effect of music on exercise adherence and treatment outcomes in a study of overweight to moderately obese women. Presented at the 2005 annual meeting of NAASO, The Obesity Society, Vancouver, October 18, 2005.

Cauza E, Hanusch-Enserer U, et al. The relative benefits of endurance and strength training on the metabolic factors and muscle function of people with type 2 diabetes mellitus. *Arch Phys Med Rehabil* 2005;86(8):1527–1533.

Elwood PC, Yarnell JW, et al. Exercise, fibrinogen, and other risk factors for ischaemic heart disease. Caerphilly Prospective Heart Disease Study. *Br Heart J* 1993;69(2):183–187.

Franco OH, de Laet C, et al. Effects of physical activity on life expectancy with cardiovascular disease. *Arch Intern Med* 2005;165(20):2355–2360.

Ham SA, Epping J. Dog walking and physical activity in the United States. *Prev Chronic Dis* 2006;3(2):A47.

Jae SY, Fernhall B, et al. Effects of lifestyle modifications on C-reactive protein: Contribution of weight loss and improved aerobic capacity. *Metabolism* 2006;55(6):825–831.

Kelley GA, Kelley KS, et al. Walking, lipids, and lipoproteins: A meta-analysis of randomized controlled trials. *Prev Med* 2004;38(5):651–661.

Lemaitre RN, Siscovick DS, et al. Leisure-time physical activity and the risk of primary cardiac arrest. *Arch Intern Med* 1999;159(7):686–690.

Noda H, Iso H, et al. Walking and sports participation and mortality from coronary heart disease and stroke. *J Am Coll Cardiol* 2005;46(9):1761–1767.

O'Donovan G, Owen A, et al. Changes in cardiorespiratory fitness and coronary heart disease risk factors following 24 wk of moderate- or high-intensity exercise of equal energy cost. *J Appl Physiol* 2005;98(5):1619–1625.

Okura T, Nakata Y, et al. Effects of exercise intensity on physical fitness and risk factors for coronary heart disease. *Obes Res* 2003;11(9):1131–1139.

Petersen AM, Pedersen BK. The anti-inflammatory effect of exercise. *J Appl Physiol* 2005;98(4):1154–1162.

Roberts CK, Barnard RJ. Effects of exercise and diet on chronic disease. *J Appl Physiol* 2005;98(1):3–30.

Serpell J. Beneficial effects of pet ownership on some aspects of human health and behaviour. *J R Soc Med* 1991;84(12):717–720.

Slentz CA, Aiken LB, et al. Inactivity, exercise and visceral fat. STRRIDE: A randomized, controlled study of exercise intensity and amount. *J Appl Physiol* 2005;99(4):1613–1618.

Stefanick ML, Mackey S, et al. Effects of diet and exercise in men and postmenopausal women with low levels of HDL cholesterol and high levels of LDL cholesterol. *N Engl J Med* 1998;339(1):12–20.

Sturm R, Cohen DA. Suburban sprawl and physical and mental health. *Public Health* 2004;118(7):488–496.

Tanasescu M, Leitzmann MF, et al. Physical activity in relation to cardiovascular disease and total mortality among men with type 2 diabetes. *Circulation* 2003;107(19):2435–2439.

Taylor RS, Brown A, et al. Exercise-based rehabilitation for patients with coronary heart disease: Systematic review and meta-analysis of randomized controlled trials. *Am J Med* 2004;116(10):682–692.

STEP 3
Getting the Right Diagnostic Tests

Austin MA, King MC, et al. Atherogenic lipoprotein phenotype: A proposed genetic marker for coronary heart disease risk. *Circulation* 1990;82(2):495–506.

McCully KS. Vascular pathology of homocysteinemia: Implications for the pathogenesis of arteriosclerosis. *Am J Pathol* 1969;56(1):111–128.

Nagai Y, Metter EJ, et al. Increased carotid artery intimal-medial thickness in asymptomatic older subjects with exercise-induced myocardial ischemia. *Circulation* 1998;98(15):1504–1509.

Ridker PM. Evaluating novel cardiovascular risk factors: Can we better predict heart attacks? *Ann Intern Med* 1999;130(11):933–937.

Shin JH, Shiota T, et al. False-positive exercise echocardiograms: Impact of sex and blood pressure response. *Am Heart J* 2003;146(5):914–919.

Stratton IM, Adler AI, et al. Association of glycaemia with macrovascular and microvascular complications of type 2 diabetes (UKPDS 35): Prospective observational study. *BMJ* 2000;321(7258):405–412.

Tsimikas S, Brilakis ES, et al. Oxidized phospholipids, Lp(a) lipoprotein, and coronary artery disease. *N Engl J Med* 2005;353(1):46–57.

Wong YK, Dawkins S, et al. Improving the positive predictive value of exercise testing in women. *Heart* 2003;89(12):1416–1421.

STEP 4
Getting the Right Medications

Arnold JM, Yusuf S, et al. Prevention of heart failure in patients in the Heart Outcomes Prevention Evaluation (HOPE) Study. *Circulation* 2003;107(9):1284–1290.

Bakris GL, Fonseca V, et al. Metabolic effects of carvedilol vs metoprolol in patients with type 2 diabetes mellitus and hypertension: A randomized controlled trial. *JAMA* 2004;292(18):2227–2236.

Barnett AH. The role of angiotensin II receptor antagonists in the management of diabetes. *Blood Press Suppl* 2001;1:21–26.

Bloomfield HE. The role of fibrates in a statin world. *Arch Intern Med* 2006;166(7):715–716.

Bonaa KH, Njolstad I, et al. Homocysteine lowering and cardiovascular events after acute myocardial infarction. *N Engl J Med* 2006;354(15):1578–1588.

Bosch J, Lonn E, et al. Long-term effects of ramipril on cardiovascular events and on diabetes: Results of the HOPE study extension. *Circulation* 2005;112(9):1339–1346.

Brown BG, Zhao XQ, et al. Simvastatin and niacin, antioxidant vitamins, or the combination for the prevention of coronary disease. *N Engl J Med* 2001;345(22): 1583–1592.

Drug interactions with grapefruit juice. *Obstet Gynecol* 2005;105(2):429–431.

Dusitanond P, Eikelboom JW, et al. Homocysteine-lowering treatment with folic acid, cobalamin, and pyridoxine does not reduce blood markers of inflammation, endothelial dysfunction, or hypercoagulability in patients with previous transient ischemic attack or stroke: A randomized substudy of the VITATOPS trial. *Stroke* 2005;36(1):144–146.

Final report on the aspirin component of the ongoing Physicians' Health Study. Steering Committee of the Physicians' Health Study Research Group. *N Engl J Med* 1989;321(3):129–135.

Haffner SM. Secondary prevention of coronary heart disease: The role of fibric acids. *Circulation* 2000;102(1):2–4.

HOPE Study Investigators. The HOPE (Heart Outcomes Prevention Evaluation) Study: The design of a large, simple randomized trial of an angiotensin-converting enzyme inhibitor (ramipril) and vitamin E in patients at high risk of cardiovascular events. *Can J Cardiol* 1996;12(2):127–137.

Joint British Societies' Guidelines on Prevention of Cardiovascular Disease in Clinical Practice. *Heart* 2005; 91: Supplement J.

Kuster GM, Amann FW, et al. High density-lipoprotein subfractions of patients using cardio-selective beta-blockers. *Cardiovasc Drugs Ther* 2002;16(2):127–131.

Liberopoulos EN, Tsouli S, et al. Preventing type 2 diabetes in high risk patients: An overview of lifestyle and pharmacological measures. *Curr Drug Targets* 2006;7(2):211–228.

Lichtenstein AH, Deckelbaum RJ. Stanol/sterol ester-containing foods and blood cholesterol levels: A statement for healthcare professionals from the Nutrition Committee of the Council on Nutrition, Physical Activity, and Metabolism of the American Heart Association. *Circulation* 2001;103(8):1177–1179.

The Lipid Research Clinics Coronary Primary Prevention Trial. Results of 6 years of post-trial follow-up. The Lipid Research Clinics Investigators. *Arch Intern Med* 1992;152(7):1399–1410.

Miller ER 3rd, Pastor-Barriuso R, et al. Meta-analysis: High-dosage vitamin E supplementation may increase all-cause mortality. *Ann Intern Med* 2005;142(1):37–46.

Nissen SE, Nicholls SJ, et al. Effect of very high-intensity statin therapy on regression of coronary atherosclerosis: The ASTEROID Trial. *JAMA* 2006;295(13):1556–1565.

Nissen SE, Tuzcu EM, et al. Effect of intensive compared with moderate lipid lowering therapy on progression of coronary atherosclerosis: A randomized controlled trial. *JAMA* 2004;291(9):1071–1080.

Paine MF, Widmer W. A furanocoumarin-free grapefruit juice establishes furanocoumarins as the mediators of the grapefruit juice-felodipine interaction. *Am J Clin Nutr* 2006;83(5)1097–1105.

Ridker PM, Cook NR, et al. A randomized trial of low-dose aspirin in the primary prevention of cardiovascular disease in women. *N Engl J Med* 2005;352(13):1293–1304.

Rundek T, Naini A, et al. Atorvastatin decreases the coenzyme Q_{10} level in the blood of patients at risk for cardiovascular disease and stroke. *Arch Neurol* 2004;61(6):889–892.

Shepherd J, Packard CJ, et al. Effects of nicotinic acid therapy on plasma high density lipoprotein subfraction distribution and composition and on apolipoprotein A metabolism. *J Clin Invest* 1979;63(5):858–867.

Taylor AJ, Sullenberger LE, et al. Arterial Biology for the Investigation of the Treatment Effects of Reducing Cholesterol (ARBITER) 2: A double-blind, placebo-controlled study of extended-release niacin on atherosclerosis progression in secondary prevention patients treated with statins. *Circulation* 2004;110(23):3512–3517.

Tenkanen L, Manttari M, et al. Gemfibrozil in the treatment of dyslipidemia: An 18-year mortality follow-up of the Helsinki Heart Study. *Arch Intern Med* 2006;166(7):743–748.

Van Horn L. Fiber, lipids, and coronary heart disease. A statement for healthcare professionals from the Nutrition Committee, American Heart Association. *Circulation* 1997;95(12):2701–2704.

INDEX

Underscored page references indicate boxed text. **Boldface** references indicate illustrations and photographs.

263

in prediabetes, 46, 74
Gopten, 228
Grains, whole. *See* Whole grains
Grapefruit, for lowering LDL cholesterol, 142
Grapefruit juice, interacting with
    medications, 142, <u>220</u>
Gruentzig, Andreas, 25

H

Haemoglobin A1c test, 207–8
Haemorrhagic stroke, 244
Hardening of the arteries. *See*
    Atherosclerosis
HDL-Atherosclerosis Treatment Study
    (HATS), 222
HDL cholesterol
  cardiac risk and, 50–51
  description of, 63, 142
  factors decreasing
    beta-blockers, 230
    diabetes and prediabetes, 46
  factors increasing
    diet, 51, 52, 142–43, 202
    exercise, 51, 142, 173, 202
    fibrates, 224
    medications, 51, 202, 218, 221, 223
    oestrogen, <u>42</u>
    smoking cessation, 51, 202
    weight loss, 51, 137, 142, 202
  guidelines for, 50, <u>65</u>, 202
  low, high triglycerides and, 143
  patient case history of, 119, 122
  in prediabetes, 74
HDL particle size
  increasing, 68, 219, 221, 224
  significance of, 62, 65, 66, **67**, 67–68, 73
  test revealing, 204–5
Healer's vs. plumber's approach to heart
    disease, 8–10, 17–21, **22–23**, 24–30
Health-care system
  financial strain on, 10
Health insurance
  tests not covered by, 88–89, 197
Heart
  anatomy and functioning of, 16–17, **18**
  natural bypasses of, 29, 112, 116, 119
Heart attack(s)
  aspirin during, 232, 241
  Calcium Score as predictor of, 4, 28, 50,
    70, <u>90</u>
  causes of, 7, 8–9, 17–20, **22–23**, 27–28,
    <u>181</u>
  definition of, 17
  emergency plan for, 239

family history of, 31
in healthy people, 15–16, 26–27, 81–82,
  197
incidence of, 7
intimal medial thickness as predictor of,
  214, 222
lipoprotein (a) and, 69
patient case histories of, 123–24
preventability of, 3–4, 5–6, 126, 218
prevention of
  with ACE inhibitors, 227, 228
  aggressive, 5–6, 8, 9, 241
  with angioplasty vs. medical therapy,
    109
  with aspirin, 231–32
  with beta-blockers, 229
  with calcium channel blockers, 230
  with cholesterol-lowering drugs, <u>13</u>,
    218, 219, 224–25
  failure of, 5, 6–8
  with fish oil, 234–35
  vs. intervention for, 8–10
  with Mediterranean diet, 136
  treatment for, 3–4, 41, 222
seeking medical help for, 122, 124,
  241–42
stroke risk after, 242
symptoms of, 239, 240–41
in women, 31, <u>43</u>, 240, 242
Heart disease. *See also* Atherosclerosis;
    Coronary artery disease
death rate from, 7
diagnosing (*see* Diagnostic tests)
hormone replacement therapy and,
  <u>42–43</u>
interventional vs. preventive approach to,
  8–10, 17–21, **22–23**, 24–30
  cardiologist's account of, <u>12–14</u>
  cost of, 10
  economic incentives for, 10
  problems with, 21, 24–27
medications for (*see* Medications)
prevention of
  former lack of, 31
  researchers in, viii–x
  role of foods in, 138–46
  with South Beach Heart Programme
    (*see* South Beach Heart Programme)
risk factors for (*see* Risk factors for heart
    disease)
role of belly fat and diabetes in, 71, 72–75
  (*see also* Belly fat; Diabetes;
    Prediabetes)
treating, with invasive procedures,
  107–24

Heart failure. *See also* Heart attack
  definition of, 17
  from high blood pressure, 48
  medications for, 227–28, 229
Heart Outcomes Prevention Evaluation
        (HOPE) trial, 227, 233
Heart Protection Study, 99, 233
Heart rate
  calculating maximum, 177–78
  medications lowering, 178, 230
Heart recovery rate, 179
Heart scan
  Calcium Score from, 4, 28, 61, 84, 90,
        208, 209–10
  contrast dye allergy and, 209
  vs. conventional cholesterol profile, 61
  cost of, 89, 92
  description of, 208–10
  for diagnosing heart disease, 30, 70, 82,
        84–85, 88, 92, 198
  history of Calcium Score and, 86–87
  for monitoring response to medications,
        92–93
  in patient case histories, 113, 115, 116,
        117, 121
  as patient motivator, 92–93, 93, 105, 198,
        210
  reliability of, 62
  schedule for repeating, 210
  when to have, 50, 88, 89
Heart screening tests, conventional,
        inadequacy of, 92
Heel Beat Variation, 191–192, **191–192**
Hennekens, Charles, 231
High blood pressure
  definition of, 47
  with diabetes, 46, 47
  haemorrhagic stroke from, 244
  as heart disease risk factor, 47–49
  from inactivity, 171
  incidence of, 47
  lowering, 49, 137, 144–46
  low-fat dairy products preventing,
        139–40, 145
  medications for (*see* Blood pressure
        medications)
  patient stories about, 44, 164–65
  with prediabetes, 74
  salt sensitivity and, 145
  thick heart muscle with, 213–4
High-sensitivity C-reactive protein
        (Hs-CRP) test, 56, 206–7
History of heart disease, as risk factor, 40–41
HMG-CoA reductase inhibitors. *See* Statins
Homocysteine

effect of B vitamins on, 55–56, 207, 233
effect of specific foods on, 56
elevated, as heart disease risk factor,
        55–56, 207
Homocysteine test, 207
HOPE trial, 227, 233
Hormone replacement therapy (HRT),
        health risks from, 42–43, 245
HRT. *See* Hormone replacement therapy
Hs-CRP test, 56, 206–7
Hydrochlorothiazide, 228
Hypertension. *See also* High blood pressure
  malignant, 49
Hypoglycaemia, reactive, 73, 77

I

Inactivity
  contributors to, 171–72, 181
  health effects of, 170–71
  as heart disease risk factor, 57–58, 167
Inderal, 229
Inflammation
  CRP as marker of, 41, 56–57, 79,
        206–7
  foods promoting, 57
  health effects from, 56, 79, 206
  from inactivity, 171
  reducing or preventing, with
    alpha-linolenic acid, 144
    loss of belly fat, 138
    monounsaturated fats, 142
    statins, 219
Insulin resistance, 72–73. *See also* Diabetes;
        Prediabetes
  from fat storage, 76, 77
  fibre preventing, 77
Interventional approach to heart disease
  economic incentives for, 10
  vs. preventive approach, 8–10, 17–21,
        22–23, 24–30
  cardiologist's account of, 12–14
Invasive heart procedures
  angioplasty, **22**, 108–10 (*see also*
        Angioplasty)
  bypass surgery, **22**, 110, 111 (*see also*
        Bypass surgery)
  complications of, 111, 117
  false promise of, 21, 24–25
  indications or contraindications, 107
    acute symptoms, 122–24
    mild chronic symptoms, 117–20
    moderate to severe symptoms,
        120–22
    no or atypical symptoms, 112–17